HELLO,

my name is NOT cancer

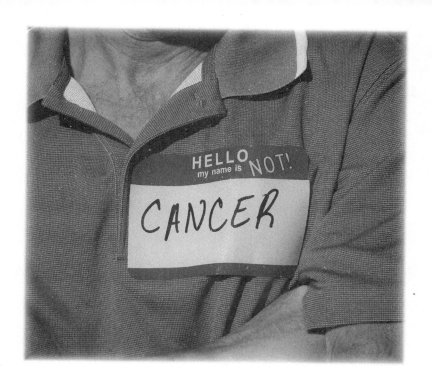

ONE MAN'S UNCENSORED
LOOK AT LIFE,
DEATH, AND IDENTITY

—Guy Beck

Huff Publishing Associates /
Quill House Publishers

MINNEAPOLIS

HELLO, MY NAME IS NOT CANCER
One Man's Uncensored Look at Life, Death, and Identity

Publishing consultant: Huff Publishing Associates, LLC
Cover and book design: Hillspring Books, Inc.

ISBN 978-1-933794-57-0

CONTENTS

Foreword   9

1   How Did I Ever Get Here?   11

2   Those Infamous Nodules   17

3   Why ME?   27

4   Back When I Thought Life Was Normal   35

5   One Evening with Death   45

6   Exposing . . . a Mission?   49

7   Let the Games Begin   57

8   Ever Want to Be a Cow?   81

9   Perceptions   83

10   To My Shame   91

11   Liz Speaks Out   95

12   600 BCE   99

13   It's Never Over When It's Over   101

14   When It's NO Fun Anymore   119

15   The Face of Grace   135

16   What Is It This Time?!   139

17 Poster Boy   145

18 Time Has a Way of Changing Your Thinking   153

19 Life and Living, Death and Dying   161

20 There Probably Is NO Good Way to Say This   167

21 Who Do You Think You Are?   175

Postscript   187

WITH A SPECIAL LOVE AND GRATITUDE
I DEDICATE THIS BOOK...

To my wife Liz who understands what it means when you vow,
"For better and for worse," and to our son Daniel,
who quietly keeps watch over our family.

To the wonderful Doctors and staff at both Loyola Medical Center,
Maywood, Illinois and Rush-Copley Medical Center, Aurora, Illinois
for the role each has played in a much larger plan; thank God.

To the members of the Sixty-second Christian Writer's Conference
in Green Lake, Wisconsin. With special thanks to John
Lehman who asked me if there was a story I needed to tell.
His help and insights propelled this work into a reality.

And, to the countless ones like me who want to be
no more than who we are!

FOREWORD

Once or twice in your life (if you're lucky) you'll find your-self watching a movie whose characters or situations resemble your own, and you want to know what's going to happen, not because it's a good movie, but because you want to know what's going to happen to you in your own life. Or maybe it's a book you read that perfectly fits your frame of mind at the time: *Catcher in the Rye* or *On the Road* or *Zen and the Art of Motorcycle Maintenance* or . . .

Well, this is my story. I was giving a writing workshop. A week or two before, I had been diagnosed with prostate can-cer. I didn't tell many people outside of my immediate fam-ily. I just didn't know how to react to the news myself. Up to this point I had lived in a world of dreams, of goals, of things I wanted to write. Into this workshop, Guy Beck came.

I think he had intended to write about something else, but one of my initial questions to the group was: "What is something that matters to you—something that you can't let go of or won't let go of you until you push everything aside and deal with it? That something is what I want you to work on this week." Guy started talking about his experiences with cancer. More than anything else, he showed "attitude." This was a person who refused to be defined by any disease. And I thought to myself, "yeah!"

Over the next few months, he sent me parts of this book. It would foreshadow what I, on a lesser level, was about to go through. And I felt there was not only someone on my side, but someone who was shouting, "Just because you're sick, you don't have to take this sitting down." Let me add, there were people who I thought would be there for me—family, friends, business associates. For one reason or another, they stood back. Now I realize it was because of fear, fear of their own mortality. It is easier to point a finger, for them to feel somehow you are to blame, and to feel "I am not like you."

At the time, I felt lonely. Except for Guy. He was my "bridge over troubled water."

I don't know if I have written like this about anything I have ever read before. Nor do I ever want to do it again. But at that turning point in my life when I most needed it, this book and Guy were there. There for me. And sure, some anger, some "attitude," could be toned down, but what Guy gives to you, reading this right now, is real. It is the thing you need the most, no matter what. It is the courage to be yourself.

—John Lehman, founder of *Rosebud Magazine*
and literary editor of *Wisconsin People & Ideas*

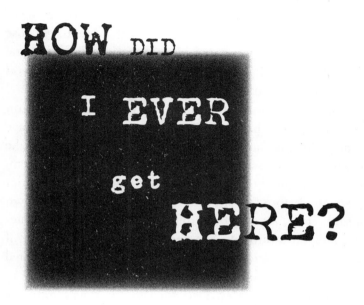

Chapter 1

HOW DID I EVER get HERE?

August 25, 2010

Ring-ring . . . Ring-ring. It was our home phone.

"Hello."

"Hello, may I speak to Guy Beck, please?"

"Ahh . . . No, this is his son Dan. He's not home at the moment. Can I take a message?"

"Yes. This is Cindy calling from the Cancer Center. Can you please have him call me as soon as possible! The number here is area code 708-_ _ _-_ _ _ _. Thank you, good bye."

The wonders of technology today—call waiting, call forwarding, and caller ID. Don't you just love it? We hang up on numbers we don't know, and we choose not to answer some of the ones we do know. How about a phone that identifies those calls you'd just as soon not get? How about inventing a phone that can tell you what the person is going to say before you answer it? How about that?!

Sometimes I come home from work to a message lying on the kitchen table. That's where we put notes we wish to leave each other, like if Dan will be late for dinner, or in cases like this, when someone calls and you need to get back to them. But it really wasn't necessary to leave a note on this particular day, because before I could catch my breath or even sit down Dan said, "Hey, Dad, Cindy from the Loyola Cancer Center called. She left a number. She needs you to call her." And if that wasn't notification enough, as soon as my wife stepped into the room she told me the same thing.

So much for the "Hey, Dad" or the "How was your day dear?" with a kiss. Cardinal Bernadine Cancer Center of Loyola Medical Center needed calling. This was all any of us needed to hear for everything else in our world to come to a screeching halt. Nothing short of death trumped an unscheduled call from Loyola. So there we all stood, each with our own brand of stuff running through our heads. Dan, wanting to relay the message promptly, hit me with it just as I walked in the door. And Liz, she might as well have just handed me the phone with the number already dialed and ringing. A prompt call back was all she needed—but didn't need, you understand.

If we share nothing else, we share the unexpected nature of life, don't we? As for me, I just wanted to catch my breath. But a sense of urgency hovered over an otherwise uneventful day, so I grabbed the paper with the number on it and headed off to our bedroom. Sometimes I'll use that phone so I can close the door so it's quieter when calling someone back, so I can hear better in case it's noisy on the other end. You know, those "special times."

Over time you come to learn a few things about the medical world. When they want to change your appointment, they send a card. And often without asking, I might add. As if our time really doesn't matter. Who can't just change their day willy-nilly? Of course, I don't mind. I only set the first appointment for a certain day and time for reasons of my own. Who cares that the day I picked just goes right out the window? Of course I don't mind just letting you pick the day and time that works best for the doctor. None of us complain. Maybe they do it to break our will. You know, we'll be better patients for it. Right? Maybe they do it because we are just a slot on a giant roulette wheel called an appointment book.

Sometimes I remind myself they are watching out for me the best they can. There is no shortage of patients at the Cancer Center. Every day the waiting room is full. Every day brings another steady stream of patients. No end in sight. What must it be like to live in Cancer Center world?

Another thing I've learned is that when test results are OK, they DON'T ask you to call back ASAP! After a while you learn to adapt to this environment. Like a chameleon you adapt; you change to fit. It's a matter of survival.

Oh, one last thing, and the most important. When they call and say they need to speak with you and leave a number, it is NEVER GOOD. So, there I am. Jammed right there in that place. So too, is my wife of 26 years, Liz, and son Dan, age 22. Like it or not, they too have some experience with all of this by now; collateral damage I suppose. Suddenly, it feels like the ugly tentacles of all this crap stretch for miles. So I make the call only to be told she has left for the day.

So you go to sleep that night knowing that sometime tomorrow you need to call the hospital back. It's interesting how you start reorganizing your day, or planning just when you might call back—as if you have a choice. That's funny.

I wanted to know if any of you ever chose not to call? Did you have any luck with that? My avoidance has never brought me healing. Did you ignore the call, and were you suddenly OK? Just wondering; that's all.

I slept fine, just in case you were wondering. By now these things don't keep me up. I believe they are outside my sphere of control. I leave them to a higher power.

The morning dawns and I head off to work. But it is still lurking in the dark parts of your brain—"I wonder what this is all about this time?" See, this is not the first time. By now, it's the third.

At work I find a quiet place and make the call. I work for Public Works; our garage can be noisy. A woman answers. I say, "Hello this is Guy Beck, Cindy asked me to return her call."

"OK, Mr. Beck, let me get her for you."

Music comes over your phone. Personally I couldn't care less. It's not as if it makes me forget who I'm waiting for on the other end. I wonder, is the music supposed to make us feel better, or distract us?

I wait. I flash back to what I have seen going on in the Cancer Center world when I've been there. I know they're busy. But they're the ones that just interrupted my life, so turnabout is fair play, right? Let's just leave it right there.

I look at my phone. Another wonder of technology—it keeps track of just how long I have been on hold. It lets me know just how much of my day has slipped out of my hands. It pisses me off that I have to make the call in the first place, let alone wait. I hang up. Screw them. I'm tired of waiting. I'm in control here! So I hang up in disgust!

An hour or so goes by and I call again. I know I'm going to call. What choice do I have? The same woman answers, or at least I think so. When I told her again who I was she seemed to remember. "Wait just a moment and I'll get her." That sounded more promising. The wait this time was shorter.

"Hello, is this Mr. Beck?"

"Yes."

"Mr. Beck can you tell me your date of birth please?"

"7-21-57."

"It looks like you had a follow-up CT last week."

"Yes."

"Well, it appears you have some nodules in your lungs. You seem to have always had nodules, but we found some new ones. Is there any chance we can move your appointment up a week?"

Now what in the world did she think I would say? Can you tell me that? It's like we play this little game. They ask nicely, we say yes, and all the while they are not really asking. So, plans you had no longer exist or get moved. Instead of going in two weeks for your routine follow-up, you get to go a week sooner. Lately, I've been going alone. It's been seven years now. This time my wife will be going! Who needs a job when we can fill our days with visits to the hospital? A job just gets in the way of all the appointments anyway. My "new" appointment time is 11:50 AM, August 27, 2010. It seems I've been at this forever.

Chapter 2

Those Infamous Nodules

Today Liz and I would be heading to Loyola to find out what that phone call was all about.

Calls like these are always disruptive. They clutter your mind with more questions. Questions left unanswered until your follow-up appointment. Planned appointments are good, but a deviation from the plan makes Liz worry and me wonder. And all it takes is just one test, that one test which comes on the heels of countless other normal tests and your mind spins, your BP goes up, and your sleep finds a few more interruptions. Status quo equals a win. All you're looking for is status quo. I never thought that "status quo" would be my new understanding of winning.

Liz never liked these follow-up appointments that came after testing. She had not gone to many of the appointments, but it's not because she doesn't care. I usually told her it's not necessary, because they'd been going along with no need for concern for years by now. I admit I was concerned, because they never move up your appointment for nothing. Yes, even after all this, some days just put you a little off your game. This appointment was different, and Liz was not about to stay home. "And the two shall become one flesh."

Long story short, in time the nurse called my name, "Mr. Beck." The usual pleasantries were exchanged. Liz followed behind as we walked down the hall. Our minds were working as we entered the exam room. We both sat down, I on the exam table and Liz in a chair along the wall. The nurse wanted weight and BP. She asked the usual barrage of questions, and I gave all the usual answers. We'd done this so many times by now I can do it in my sleep. The nurse made her notations on the computer, said the doctor would be in just a moment, and left the room closing the door. Liz and I exchanged only glances.

It's nice when the clinic's day is running smoothly. Guarantees our day will run smoothly as well, or at least as smooth as a visit to your friendly neighborhood Cancer Center can go. Soon there was a knock on the door, and in popped Dr. Frank. We exchanged more niceties, introductions for Liz and the doc, and he got right to it.

Dr. Frank began, "I know what you were told, but I just don't see it."

Liz exhaled an audible groan of relief. I sat there and said, "OK." There was an image on the computer screen of a section from my CT with a highlighted marker on it. Didn't look like anything to me, but who am I? I guess we were looking for some small pea shaped thing, which I couldn't find even by the marker. Dr. Frank went on to say that sometimes the sectioned images catch an edge of something or whatever, and it comes up like something "new." I assure you he used more technical language, but "something" and "whatever" work for our discussion.

So there we sat. Relieved, more at ease, wondering what all the fuss was about. I thought, "Well, if it's nothing, then what in the heck am I doing here a week early? Why freak out my wife and me and then tell me I'm OK? This all seems very unnecessary. Why?" But then, there was a part of me that didn't care about all the tension or anxiety these visits can cause. I didn't care because good results are good, no matter how you get the news.

Results good or bad always produce one thing: more questions. You might not think it should work that way, but it does. I always find myself asking, "So what's next?"

Dr. Frank was quick to answer my "what's next" question. He made two suggestions. First, I was to go and see a pulmonologist (lung guy). He felt very confident about the scans, but not so confident apparently to just cut me loose. He said that the lungs were not his specialty and suggested it would be good to have my CT checked by a specialist. Who can argue with that? It's not like you want to let it go, as if lung nodules are no big deal.

Second, he suggested that we see each other again in three months. I had been thinking August per our usual schedule. Not this time. He offered three or four months and then settled on three. I agreed. After all, he's the doctor. He said he would feel better if he saw me in three. OK, visit over. He updated my orders and asked me to get blood work done as part of the three-month recheck. He was polite and headed off to the next guy.

At the counter we made two appointments this time, one for the pulmonologist and one for the three-month follow-up.

That was that. We both walked out a few pounds lighter that day. Invisible weight is still weight.

TIME HAPPENS

The three months passed quickly. I almost forgot about the recheck. It's not like I didn't remember, but I actually forgot for a while. Once in a while it is nice to forget. It was June 9, 2011, the night before the follow-up CT scan to confirm once more that I either did or did not have new nodules in my lungs. It was another typical day at work; I did my thing and headed home rather than go to my dad's. My mom just passed away some months earlier, and I liked to go see my dad just to make sure he was OK, but time made other demands of my day. I had some phone calls to make regarding Dad's affairs, now that Mom was gone. Revelation: there is only so much time in the day. A lesson I am still learning. So there I was running a list in my head as I drove home. Whom do I need to call, and in what order? I got home, cleaned up things from my lunch bag, took off my work clothes in the bedroom, and noticed we had three messages on the answering machine. So I hit the button. The first two are junk calls and then a nice sounding man comes on to remind me I have a 7 AM CAT scan appointment tomorrow. I listen to the reminder and reach for my papers and bottle of barium. Yep, there it was: Friday, June 10, 2011, 7 AM.

Just like that. Remember how I said these things have a way of catching us off guard? So I picked up the bedside phone and called my boss. I got his answering machine. I told him in the message that I couldn't come in for work at seven because I would be at Loyola for another test. I said I would be in as soon as the test is done. Just like that. What are they going to say? And, it's not like I'm going to miss the appointment. That would only mess up the follow-up with the doc.

That's not going to happen. Thankfully, I have a boss and a job that allows for these things to happen without fallout. Thank God.

It's about 9:30 PM. I just got done mixing and drinking my bedtime barium cocktail. My wife commented that one day I was just going to start glowing, and my son looked at me and said, "Down the hatch!" Sooner or later everyone gets in on the fun.

That night, it wasn't so pleasant to get down. I was glad that half was done. Five AM would be round two, the second two cups of barium mixture. Zowie! I could hardly wait. Ah, the tests aren't bad; it's just drinking this stuff that's lousy. You test and wait at least a week for the results; right now I don't remember the exact date for the follow-up with the doctor. Oh well, I'll figure it out, or they'll call me again to remind me. That's the routine; test and wait.

The follow-up appointment with the doctor was June 16th. That gave us plenty of time to wait on the outcome once again. Isn't life wonderful? Begs the question doesn't it: will you let the waiting bother you?

Let's try something different on for size. How would you respond to the question, "What are you thankful for?" Are you thankful that we have CT technology? Are you thankful that you just had one? I asked the radiologist how many I have had, if she knew. She said, "I only have the short list since 2006; you have had six to date." But, that was the short list. This all began in 2004. Years one and two probably equal six or seven, so we're probably up to twelve or thirteen.

I digress, but did you know that runners or tri-athletes put distance numbers on the back window of their cars? (By the way, this is something I have never done, and don't plan on doing anytime soon.) Like someone behind you will oooh or ahhh as they read it. Maybe we could start something new and put our CT numbers on our back window? What do you think? My total number of CT scans just jumped up one, a new personal record!

The truth is the results of my test today are already in. I don't know them yet. Quite probably they have not been read yet even by the radiologist. But they're in, new nodules or not, and right now I am living in one reality or the other without so much as a clue. So, why waste time worrying or wondering. Time will only confirm what my body and the Almighty already know.

It was both funny and ironic that day. I had just sat down in the waiting area when over the speaker system came the retro Abba song, "SOS," which is, of course, understood to be the international code for distress. Hospital—SOS, I chuckled, and noted it in my head. It's OK to chuckle. I chuckled first so go right ahead, you have my permission, should you need it. It doesn't bother me if you laugh. Please, scratch your head, think its weird, smile or laugh—really, it's OK. But, just so you know, I won't be downloading SOS to my play list anytime soon.

The appointment that day went off smoothly. Not a long wait. Greeted the woman at the desk; gave her my name, date of birth, and appointment time—that's protocol. I took my seat in the waiting area. Right on time a nice nurse called my name. As I approached she commented, "You knew you were next didn't you?" I said "yes," and we headed to Room A3. It was the eye contact. I just knew when we made eye contact before she called my name that I would be next.

With that we entered the exam room, and she took my weight and blood pressure; the BP was a little high again. She asked about it and wondered if it was only because I was coming here. I told her it had been running a little high, but maybe even subconsciously my body was reacting to all the junk hanging in the air. Her eyes seemed sympathetic as she nodded. She asked the standard set of questions and then said, "You've done this before, haven't you?"

"Yes," I said and added, "for quite some time by now."

Next she asked if I could give her a urine sample. I assured her I could, so she gave me the standard sample kit, an alcohol swab in a sealed little packet, and a plastic jar with a sealed lid in a larger plastic bag. Off I went, heading down the hall to the bathrooms. I'm not inviting you in.

As I arrived at the bathrooms another gentleman approached as well. He got there first and checked both handles. They were both being used. So, me being me, I said, "Full house." The other guy replied, "I guess so." That was it. We stood there in the hall with our clear plastic jars and our bag and swab. Again, I can't tell you how many samples I have given by now, but that day it felt awkward. It just did. I can't tell you what he was thinking; I just looked around as if casually interested in my surroundings and left that right there. There we were, that other guy and I. It felt like all kinds of unspoken junk was swirling round in both our heads. Weird, I know. Once it was my turn, I did the deed and put the specimen in the small metal enclosure in the wall of the bathroom used to collect these things and headed back to the room.

Once back to the room I sat and waited for the doctor. While I waited I heard Dr. Frank in the hall direct a nurse to make sure and schedule Mr. So and So. I didn't catch his name, and wouldn't tell you anyway, for a prostate biopsy. That kind of sent a shiver through me. I was thinking, I've been at this for six and a half years now, and he's just getting started.

In time, Dr. Frank walked in. We did all of the usual physical examinations. He commented that I looked great and asked if I was still running. Then he got right to the results. Everything looks stable, no new nodules present. This test removed all of the doubts from the last. That was his diagnosis! I could still hear his words from the last questionable test, "I just don't see it!" The results of the chest/thorax with contrast CT showed no changes. The nodules that are present in my lungs had not changed. I quote from patient information sheet: "FINDINGS: There is no thoracic lymphadenopathy. No pleural or pericardial effusion. The four previously identified bilateral lung nodules (images 9, 25, 30) are stable. There are no new lung nodules. There is a stable splenula. IMPRESSION: < 5 MM lung nodules are stable since 8/12/10. There are no new abnormalities." Just kind of rolls off the tongue, doesn't it? All kinds of details that can be summed up in two words, "Good News."

It really struck me that the clinic was like a bee hive, filled with doctors, interns, nurses, administrative staff—and us drones. We come when called. We do as ordered. In and out we go. The Cancer Center never seems to be at a loss for patients.

When I got a copy of the results in the exam room I said thank you under my breath. The thank you was not intended for the doctor. It wasn't an exuberant "thank you," just a "thank you." It's not that I didn't care, or wasn't incredibility grateful, because I was. But, there are times when quiet forms of gratitude are all you can muster. A sigh, a lowering of the head, a whispered, "Thank you," each a singular form of thanks offered in the world of perceived blessings. There have been a lot of signs of gratitude over these many years. That day it was a quietly whispered, "Thank you."

I walked out to my car and drove home, just kind of in a flat sort of a way. I called Liz first to let here know all was well, and then I also called my friend Gregg, who said, "That's good news; I've been praying about it."

That's was nice to hear. After six years, some are still interested and ask. Others I don't even keep informed anymore. I wonder if not telling some is my way of lessening what is still going on?

I told Gregg, "Add another CT to my list." Jokingly, I said, "Yeah, my prostate and testicular cancers have shown no signs of return, but now I have another cancer from the radiation I have been getting from the testing." Gregg and I laughed.

Gregg said, "Mr. Beck, I have some good news and bad. The cancers we have been treating are gone—but . . ." Then we both laughed again. One way or another it's always out there. Question is: Are you staring it down, or is it staring you down?

Once home Liz commented, "I was hoping for more than three months. I didn't want it to be only three months; I wanted it to be a year."

I told her it would be ok. She cried as she said, "Three more months of worry. I didn't want to have to worry for a year." That's how this goes. Liz told me once again, "Pretty soon you're going to glow in the dark."

I told her, "Then you won't need a flashlight." I headed for the kitchen. Liz headed for the tissue box.

See, by her way of thinking they wouldn't want me back in three months if there was really nothing to worry about. For me, doc said there is nothing new—case closed. Returning in three months will only confirm what "I" already know—nothing has changed, no new nodules. Period!

All in all it was a good day. I'm in the clear for three more months, or maybe the rest of my life—thank God. In three months, we'll get geared up and do it all over again.

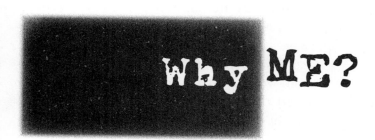

Chapter 3

Why ME?

Seems like a reasonable question, wouldn't you say?

But, that's not what I'm talking about. How about, because I feel I'm an average Joe. White collar, blue collar, I've done them both. I've both refused to attend college as a young man in favor of a job as a cabinetmaker, and also chosen later in life to attend college culminating in a Master of Divinity Degree from Northern Baptist Seminary. Both experiences helped me grow and mature as part of this journey. I especially enjoyed my years under

Northern Seminary's tutelage. They provided me with a great environment in which to come to terms with many things.

Why me? Maybe it's just because I'm willing, willing to tell the whole story, at least as far as my story goes. I'm not afraid to be open; I like being open now. Openness has become a fruit of my journey as well. Here, in these pages, I get to be open, and open is very freeing. Open is simple. How about, because I'm willing to say out loud what many are only thinking. People have thanked me for telling my story out loud, and were freed to speak because of it.

Curiosity is a trait we all share when it comes right down to it. For that reason I think there are people out there who desperately want to know how living with cancer "really" is but don't know how to ask. We are a curious people, aren't we? I think a lot of people on both sides of this issue just might benefit from some of my open honesty. I know there are others who would like to tell you their story but can't. After this, maybe they will be empowered to do so. That would be awesome.

So who am I? Nobody special, really. Nothing besides living it qualifies me to write to you about this. I grew up in middle-class America, in the suburbs. I was born in 1957 to wonderful parents, Evelyn and Harold. I have an identical twin brother. My mom was forty at the time of our birth, so we were plenty. My parents both worked. My dad is still living and will be turning eighty-eight later this year. My mom just passed away a month ago, as you already know. Mom was ninety-two. That's that. I could define for you the many specific events of our family's life, but then you'd miss the point.

It's not about how I grew up. It's not about where I lived. It's not about having a twin brother. It's not about taking care of dad, burying mom, or even what they did for a living. Oh, I know that there are genetic markers, or family histories, but really our lives are all very much the same. My life, your life, our lives are what they are. In many ways our differences unite us under the greater umbrella of cancer. The disease doesn't care that I grew up to loving parents, or lived in a nice middle-class neighborhood, or that maybe you didn't. Cancer couldn't care less that my family and I took trips to Wisconsin.

Cancer is not an opportunist. I wasn't chosen because cancer had it out for me, or because I am someone important, or that cancer saw me as a threat. Though, on second thought, maybe it should see me as the latter. It's funny. Just think of how many times celebrities are in the news especially when they are diagnosed with cancer. I never made the news—not so much as one word—nor did I care. Cancer doesn't care when you make the news. Some people struggle with cancer alone. Others have many who care, and what a blessing that is. Then there are those of us who fall somewhere in the middle. I guess that's where I have seen myself.

When I think of the monies raised, or the miles that are walked, it's awesome, but they only help the research. For many of us, that will mean very little. Research is really about the future. The hope that we can spare others from what we have had to endure drives many to find "the cure." But will those who have been spared cancer really be the better for it? I know that to remember loved ones touched by cancer gives them life again, if only briefly. And to remember them in this way brings healing but only for the living.

Why me? Maybe it's finally time to get out all that junk that has been roaming around in my being for years now. There have been so many things that surround the vast world of cancer that have frankly annoyed me. I have found the process of writing this book to be a relief, actually.

Why me? Because I needed to wake up and believe there are many out there like me. If I may be so bold as to speak for men, we not only need to wake up to cancer issues confronting men, but wake up to the fact that there are others out there who just may want us around. When you ignore the

30

obvious as I did, you have become just as ignorant as I was. Burying your head in the sand cures nothing. Playing the macho game won't kill cancer cells; it'll only kill you. Ignorance and denial are poor remedies.

The hard truth is, when we refuse to get the care or checkups we need we demonstrate only one thing—our selfishness. So maybe part of all this exposure is about some attempt at atonement. My wife and son are lucky. I'm lucky! My stupidity has caused a lot of undue pain. I came up with a lot of reasons to avoid getting checked. Please don't follow my poor example. If you're plagued by a nagging voice, then you already know what you need to do, but haven't done yet—right?

Of course, there are those times when powers greater than yourself seem to have set things in motion unbeknownst to you. For example, Liz and I found ourselves up north for the weekend with no special agenda. Liz sat at the kitchen table at my parent's summer home to read the morning paper with her coffee, and I headed off to the Baptist Conference Center in Green Lake to go for a run. The conference center is open to the public. The grounds are beautiful, some sections wooded, others open and prairie-like. When the wind blows through the white pine it just sounds wonderful. It is a wonderful place to get free from all of life's encumbrances. So, when I get the chance I like to run there.

After a couple laps around the grounds I headed back to the cottage. As soon as I walked in the door Liz told me about a Christian writer's conference being held there in August. We knew they held one there, but knew no more details than that. I commented that it sounded nice, but August was a long way off. Thinking we were finished, I started to head off to clean up, Liz stopped me and said, "You need to go to this!" It was not said as a suggestion, if you catch my drift. I told her, "That sounds good; I'll check into it." I have done a little writing over the years, and the conference seemed like a great opportunity to explore my interest in writing.

Later that evening we had dinner with long-time friends Gregg and his wife Linda. I brought up the August writing conference, and Gregg thought that it sounded interesting. He knew I enjoyed writing but had not attended a writer's conference. The next morning we headed back home to Illinois. That was that.

The next morning at work my cell phone rang. It was my friend Gregg. We talk often, but this wasn't a social call. He was calling about the writer's conference. He admitted that he too was interested in writing and that his wife Linda had already looked up the conference on the web. This was something I didn't know about Gregg. Linda knew dates, times, and costs! I was shocked. He also admitted that the week of the conference "just happened" to coincide with his vacation week, a week he had given notice for some time ago. Linda called the host person that same day. It was then that she was told that the registration had just closed, BUT if we emailed our info and sent out a check ASAP she assured us we were in. Boom. Off went the registration, check and all.

The timing was perfect, if you asked me. I had written a study guide, a small book really, for a class I teach at church and it needed some editing, critiquing, and polish. This was going to give me just that opportunity. I was excited to go. I got all my stuff in order at home and waited for the weeks to pass. Finally, the weekend of the conference arrived. It felt great to be headed up north again. Once there, I drove over to Gregg's and picked him up. We were both excited.

The first evening of the conference was brief. All of the writers met, and the hosts asked us to define our interests— fiction, non-fiction, poetry, etc. My friend Gregg headed off with the fiction group, and I headed off to the non-fiction group.

It was there I first met John Lehman, an interesting fellow, striking in manner and in his instructing of the class. We did the usual things, such a as intros, interests, and such.

Each time I got a chance to share I spoke about the book I had finished and wanted to publish. Everyone in our group was very nice, and soon the time came to wrap things up. It was then—that moment—that unexpected, unanticipated moment, when John gave us some homework. Homework. Most of us don't like homework, but I'm a fan, and after all, it was a writing conference wasn't it? But John didn't ask us to write. Instead, he asked us one question, "Is there something, anything, that you have just wanted to write about, but haven't as of yet? Come back tomorrow morning and bring with you two or three ideas, and we'll each share them with the class, and see what we (the class) think."

Suddenly my mind was filled with a string of questions: "But, what about my agenda?" "What about the book I came here to work on?" "What about that!" That was it, and we adjourned for the night. I like sticking to what I have prepared for. I like knowing what's coming and being prepared in advance. I don't often like shake-ups. As I worked it over and over in my head I thought, "Well, you're signed up for this conference, and this is what you have been asked to do. Are you going to do what you came here to do, or are you willing to play the game?" I thought, "Well, it's only one assignment, and it isn't hurting anything, so just go along and see what happens."

The next morning our group met together, something we would do each morning of the seminar. It was another opportunity, as these things go, to go around the room and share your ideas with the group. When it was my turn I spoke up, "Well, I didn't really have two or three ideas. I just kind of have one. You see I have had cancer."

Normally, I don't go out of my way to talk about my cancers. It's not been my thing. But there I was, in a room of strangers, telling them that I have had two different types of cancer, three really, and well, this whole survivor mentality just drives me nuts. I ended by saying, "I just wish I could tell people and friends to stop letting cancer rule and define your life!" This went off in the room like a bomb. Faces filled with shock dotted the room. No one, not even me, saw this coming.

I had everyone's attention. When most people get this kind of info head on, well, it's kind of like that deer in the headlights look. When you protest boldly against the "survivor" mentality, they're just not ready. They weren't, but that didn't mean they didn't find my topic interesting. John and the other participants each asked some great questions, and they seemed most curious. Day Two's assignment was to write a few pages on our topics for the next day's review and critique.

It was as if the flood gates had been opened. Verbalizing only a small part of what was inside, listening to the reactions by my colleagues—my head was whirling as I begin to recall all that I had been through, and how I could express it on paper. It was in that moment that I knew I needed to put it in writing—all of the gory details, the honest perspectives and retrospectives, where I had come, how I grew and matured, and how I was changed. Changed in a way that I believe can be helpful and freeing for others.

Feelings I had harbored and stewed over for years came to life. I knew why each of the events leading to this conference went the way they did; like a locomotive running down its track, it felt unstoppable.

So, maybe this is really about permission. John and the class members gave me permission—permission to be who I am as a cancer patient, permission to be me, Guy. For reasons I can't fully understand yet, it was easy to talk to those wonderful folks. It was easy to give our group permission to speak up, ask questions, and drill me if they wished, without fear.

See, one thing I knew for sure is that cancer touches everyone. If you have had cancer you know firsthand that our cancers touch the lives of so many others in profound ways.

In time, over years really, I discovered so many lessons to be learned. So many questions faced. There were so many people out there who wanted to know what facing cancer was like, coming with their own questions and struggles. So I wrote, and we talked, and we shared. This is what I wish to share with you as well.

Chapter 4

BACK WHEN I THOUGHT life WAS NORMAL

Boy, does this bring back memories, memories as vivid as if they happened yesterday.

It is spring/summer 2004, and I'm strolling through halls whose numbered rooms never seem to end. I am in the middle of my internship, an internship required to complete my undergraduate training in Christian Ministry.

For six months I would drive to Rush-Copley Hospital in Aurora one day a week, meeting with Chaplain Dan Sullivan. He was showing this rookie the ropes. At each meeting we would discuss current situations that may require our assistance, go over new patient info, and address any new concerns involving patients we'd visited before.

Shirt and tie, except on Fridays; white coat with Hospital insignia, name tag fully visible and badge with security stuff, pen, some of Dan's business cards should someone need to speak directly to him, and a small Bible. You're ready for the day.

The hospital layout is very sprawling. Many long corridors bisect shorter hallways set at 45 degree angles. Many of the bisecting halls open into larger areas containing a central desk and adjoining recording stations for nurses, doctors, and other staff. Busy as bees in their hive they all buzz along doing what they are supposed to do. So, too, did Dan and I.

In time I was on my own, always listening to the overhead speakers for trauma notification accompanied by the almost simultaneous beeping of my pager. Next stop, the ER. Baptism by fire,; there's really no way to prepare until you're in the middle of it. That day I sat with a nice woman and her family whose husband passed away. He was young and getting ready for a celebration. That all changed, and change didn't care. The woman's husband was here one moment and gone the next. What are we to make of times like these? I couldn't help wonder. I still can't help wonder, but I have a little bit better idea now.

As a chaplain, you give them the help you can. Sometimes you just sit there. Sometimes, I wondered in my head, "What am I really supposed to say?" Most days, though, were not spent in the ER. They were spent walking the halls, seeing patient after patient, the list received at the morning meeting.

"Knock, knock." I would generally enter the room slowly, quickly scanning the surroundings. "Hello, my name is Guy, and I'm a chaplain with the hospital. I just came by to see if there was something you might need?" In retrospect, that sounds really stupid. Here they are in a hospital, lying in a bed for some very explainable and often visible reason, and I'm asking them if they need something.

Sorry, I digress.

Each patient was asked as part of the admissions process if they had a faith preference, and what it might be if they answered yes. They can decline if they so choose, but many people did identify their faith preference by checking the appropriate box on the form. This gave me a heads up in many instances before seeing them as to how they might react to a visit from a chaplain. Early on, my eyes were limited to the visible, but over time, I could see well beyond what was only visible with the human eye. I could see a whole lot more than they may have realized. I never quite knew how these visits would go, or what to expect when I entered a room.

I remember wanting to pray with anyone who would let me. I believe there is nothing more powerful that we can do for another person than prayer. Prayer moves us from the impossibilities of earth to the measureless possibilities of heaven.

Many patients were nice. Many were nice even as they let you know that they were not interested in your prayers or help! It was one of those days. A day spent in countless knocks in expectant opportunity followed by countless "Thank you for stopping by, but no thanks." This day brought me to the end of one of the many halls and a time of looking out the window at the day.

Exactly which hall, I've forgotten now. There I was standing in my white coat, shirt and tie with accessories. Spirit downcast like my shoulders. What of my resolve? It was beautiful outside, the sun shining brightly. The stack of patient info sheets in my jacket pocket hung like a ball and chain. I can remember asking, "Why? What good is this doing anyone?" I came to pray, and see God work, not get rejected. When I left a room without permission to pray, it wasn't me they were turning their back on, though it felt like that, it was God. And if God has the power to do anything, then why in the world weren't they almost begging me to pray for them. I hated that feeling.

This day made me want to quit. I stood by the windows at the end of one of those diagonal halls staring, staring out the window contemplating what I would do next. The decision was simple: stay and continue or go home and call it a day. But there was also that still small voice asking, "But why are you here, Guy? Are you here for them, or are you here for yourself?" "I am here for them Lord; you know that." Then a voice in my head answered back, "Then stop feeling sorry for yourself and go."

There was only one more ticket left in my pocket. One more door to knock on, one more patient to see—one more. So I kicked myself in the butt and headed for that last room. It wasn't much of a walk; the window I had been standing by was just beyond that room's door. I had been right there all along.

I knocked on the door, which was half open. A technician and a nurse were working in the room. There, lying in the bed was an elderly gentleman who appeared to be nice. He could have been any of our grandfathers. He must have glanced at my jacket. That's how he knew who I was, but I didn't see it. In only seconds after my arrival he bellowed, "You're just the man I need to see! The rest of you can come back later. I need to talk to this man." It still brings tears to my eyes, and lump to my throat as I recall this. Who knows, maybe he saved my life that day. It wasn't long before he wanted me to read scripture to him and recite some of the classics; one was Psalm 23.

We talked for quite some time. He shared. I listened. To this day I don't remember the reason for his hospitalization. But I know why he was there. He was there for me. I know he ministered to me way more than I him. By the time we were done, I had told him I don't know how many times, "It was I who needed you on this day. You were sent here for me, not I for you!" He smiled. I smiled. I wished him well. We prayed. I left, but I was not the same.

By now you're probably wondering what this has to do with my cancer. Here's when things were about to change. Here is when the handwriting on the wall was going to come into focus. I find it most ironic that it began here. It's as if secretly, without my knowledge, someone was challenging God, saying, "Can the healer heal himself?" Let's see. Put him to the test and let's just see.

GUINEA PIG

"Sure why not?" Helping out is always a good thing. Who doesn't like to help out? In most cases I like being able to help. This day was no different. I was still in the midst of my internship. The lab was looking for some guinea pigs. At that time, my brother was director of the lab. So, whom do you think he would ask if they needed some test subjects? Me.

From time to time, when new products in collection are being tested they need a few willing souls. Blood doesn't bother me. Testing doesn't bother me. And why not? The lab would run the sample, and I would get the results. Kind of like a little thank you for helping out. The test they would run, a generic blood panel, sounded cool. I hadn't been to the doctor in forever, and seeing results fascinates me.

The draw went like clockwork. The lab tech put one of those rubber tourniquets around my arm and inserted the needle into a nice juicy vein prominently exposed above my arm. That was quick. A couple of vials later and it was over, no big deal. Off to my rotations I went.

Later when I saw my brother, he had the results. It was interesting. Gary and I are identical twins. He too had volunteered. So we got to see our numbers side by side. It was amazing how identical they were, especially when you consider how precise the testing is, and how down to the fractions this stuff is measured.

Problem was, one set of numbers was not the same, not identical. But, who cares that my brother's number for that specific test was .08 and my number was 1.8. Who cares? I didn't care. Why should I? Except, all of our other values were so identical it meant this was a glaring difference that I should have checked out. So, he recommended that I see a urologist associated with the hospital. For those who don't know, urologists are the doctors who deal with stuff specific to men's health, in particular male tests like PSA. Get the picture? He gave me the name of a doctor whose office was right by work. I called and made the appointment.

LITTLE DID THEY KNOW

I don't remember the exact date of the office visit following the initial testing. I'd have to look it up, but it wasn't long after, probably one week. They like to get you in quickly when they're concerned with what may be going on.

I called almost immediately because it seemed important and prudent to do so. But truthfully, I think cluttering your mind with all those dates and things just muddies the water, and you never see clear again. I kept a record of the dates of all of my doctor's appointments for a while. Then I threw the record away—maybe in the name of survival? I haven't worked that out in my head yet.

Our son Dan told us when he was young that his head contained drawers. After a while the drawers get full. If something gets added, something must go. Too many other things are way more important.

I think many medical offices are the same. Posted on the glass, usually outside the door, is a list of doctors' names. Some days all it tells me is that an invisible much longer list of names is recorded in row after row of those non-descript filing cabinets. Row after row of people's lives, identities, tales of woe and hope—all reduced to scribbling on a chart by some doctor or staff person noting our progress or decline.

Anyway, you push open the door. Chairs in neat cube-like formations follow the floor plan of the room. A counter signaling where you are to begin is often staffed by pretty young women dressed in scrubs. "Can I help you?"

You approach the counter. "Yes. My name is Mr. Beck. I have a something o'clock appointment with Dr. so-and-so." It's not like you haven't been thinking about it. Often these offices are adorned with various pieces of art, and of course the usual stack of magazines. Oh, and that same universal clipboard they all use to gather details of your life you'd really just as soon not tell anyone. Just once I would like to tell them to shove that clipboard and let them know in no uncertain terms—"I'm tired of it!" But I didn't. I took my seat like a good little boy. Filled out the clipboard and waited. In retrospect I wish I had a dollar for every one of those I have filled out. At least it would have helped defray the costs—yeah, right.

I had never been to an urologist before. I wasn't much into all that preventative health stuff. If you don't feel bad, why go? Seemed logical at the time. I think it seems logical to most of us, especially us men, at least the ones I know. I knew an examination of some kind was in order. Every doctor has some protocol that demands an examination. It all felt really kind of weird as I sat there. Then they called my name. "Mr. Beck, right this way." I sensed something lying just beneath the surface though. It was making me a little more uneasy than normal. There was something else going on that no one knew but me.

STUPID, *NOT* IGNORANT

Stupid, not ignorant; it bears repeating. There's a BIG difference. Looking back, there I was, 47 years old. Going along, job, wonderful wife and son, living out my faith, trusting in my God.

Have you ever been stupid? What about ignorant? I'm not referring to acting ignorant, which I also have done by the way; I'm referring to ignorant like when you don't know something. This time ignorance could not be blamed; I was being stupid, and stupid in the name of faith. Let me explain. At times we can make poor (stupid) choices because we are ignorant of details that would change the way we would make a decision. Sometimes we make poor (stupid) choices because they're just bad, with no real fault on our part. But, at other times our choices are really, really, stupid, and we make them consciously. We know better, repeatedly know better, and still we do the stupid thing.

Is there any person on the planet who has not heard of the disease cancer yet? Is there any person on the planet who has not heard specific warnings about certain types of cancers that can easily be detected through self-examination? GUYS, and we know who we are, have any of you guys not heard of a PSA test or not been told to do a self-examination of your testicles for testicular cancer?

A simple blood test provides us with a PSA number and you have a window into how your prostate is doing. Do a self-examination of, well you know, and if one or the other, or both seems out of shape, or has a different density, it's time to see the doctor.

So why would I make such a statement about God and stupidity and faith? What does any of that have to do with this? Everything! That's all—everything! Sometimes when you're a blockhead like me you tend to be stupid about the obvious. I had no excuse. I was well acquainted with all of the stuff that's gone on around the issue of testicle cancer. AND I chose to be stupid, and I chose to use faith to promote my stupidity.

Have you ever seen that shower scene from Psycho—hysterical screaming, followed by a horrific panicked stare?

I took my showers. Everyone takes showers. Then at some point I began to notice some changes in my left testicle and thought nothing. Down this happy little path I continued. In time being a God fearing man, I prayed. In stupidity I continued. Continued to ignore the obvious, so I prayed for healing, and continued to do nothing. The size and density differences became more obvious. I'd pray all the more—and did nothing.

I can't tell you how many times I said to myself, "Guy, you know you have testicular cancer. I can't tell you how many times a voice in my head told me, "Guy, the vast array of health info out there today has given you all the information you need to know that this is what is going on." I will even tell you that the Lord told me himself, "Guy, it's testicular cancer!" Even at that, I DID NOTHING and kept PRETENDING it was going to go away! I would even tell the Lord, "If it's going to get corrected you're going to have to be the one to do it."

I DID NOTHING BUT PRAY FOR TWO YEARS, and IT DIDN'T GO AWAY!

Don't get me wrong: I believe strongly in God's ability and willingness to heal. I have seen the healing power of prayer. But sometimes God chooses to work through mechanisms already in place, like awareness and medical personnel and common sense. Sometimes God has a different path in mind than answered prayer. Sometimes God needs to use a baseball bat, at least if you're like me.

I know that some of you right now are living only moments from God's baseball bat . . . and this may be your last answered prayer. The clock's ticking. Your shot at ignorance is running out. It's your call. So God got out a baseball bat and gave me a whack: thank God for that test and technology! There was no more time to waste. No more options. I couldn't run from this reality any longer. It was time to get checked out.

44

Trust me. You won't be sorry. How much is peace of mind worth to you? Trust me; it's better to know EVEN WHEN THE RESULTS AREN'T WHAT YOU'RE HOPING FOR. Make the call! Don't be stupid!

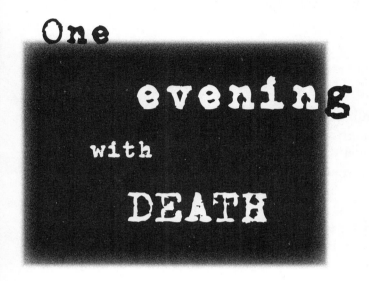

Chapter 5

One evening with DEATH

It is late fall 2001. A man sits to one end of a long plaid sofa.

He sits with his hands folded in his lap, head bowed. This is the same man who only moments or minutes earlier found himself kneeling in prayer on the basement floor. A lamp on the end table lights the room, but not brightly. It is dark outside by now. Evening is pressing on. It's fall in the Midwest. This is familiar space. Many hours have already passed in uneventfully similar fashion. Quietly he sits praying for family and friends. Quietly he thinks.

Seeks to hear. Tries to listen. It is then, in these moments that a feeling, not fully explainable, comes over the room—then the man. It is as if he is no longer alone.

✻ ✻ ✻

The retelling sends a shiver through my body, my body remembering what my mind only remembers in part now. I can tell you the man was no longer alone. Looking around the room would have produced no evidence visible to the human eye that someone had joined the man, yet there he sat right next to the man, on the plaid sofa. He sat to his left. What passed as forever I was sure was only seconds. The man's mind was working, the man's spirit was working, the Spirit was working to discern what was happening here. Then he knew, but not as old friends sharing a fresh look at a beloved friend. This night it was Death. It was Death who was paying him a visit.

The conversation that ensued was brief and one-sided. It was the man who would do all the talking. It was Death who was going to have to listen. "I don't know why you're here," the man spoke audibly to his guest, "but I know who you are. I know you're Death." There was no response. I no longer remember how long the two spoke. But the message from the man was clear, "I know you're Death, and I am not afraid! I know you have no power over me unless God says so. And—if God says so, that's OK too, because I trust him."

No raised voice. No fear. The man's only goal was to remind Death of his place, his tenuous hold on the power, which he doesn't truly have. The man knew that one day Death, too, would meet his end. He knew, and that knowledge gave him more power than Death. Exactly why Death came still remains a mystery. The message Death would receive left no vague confusions. "I know who you are! I'm not afraid of you!"

Just as suddenly as the room had changed the first time, it changed back again. The room returned to what the man had known many times before, a quiet place of prayer. I suppose the question still hangs in the air of that basement just as the sofa still sits in its old familiar place.

In retrospect I wonder: that night was he praying for what WAS or what was TO COME? Makes me think. Now I know only in part what Job must have felt like as he became a pawn in what I often refer to as a cosmic chess match between Good and Evil—God and Satan. Job was truly a righteous man. I'm no Job.

I can't say I haven't wondered from time to time how it will be when we meet again. Will there be the familiar, "Hello Death, we meet again." I expect no response. Maybe a slight nod of the head; we'll see.

One thing is clear and two things are certain: my first death will be of little consequence compared to Death's death. My heart rests safe in a sphere that lies beyond doubt. I will exhale in this life and draw a new breath with eternal hope in my next life. I will close my eyes, only for a second, opening them anew in the Kingdom of God. Death is not going to be so lucky. I hope he's really good at treading fire, and for a really long time.

And if Death is listening out there somewhere, I wish to say, "When I see you again, it will be for the last time for both of us. Your days are coming to end, and you can't do a _____ thing about it! Thanks to MY Jesus!"

As I have had opportunity to look back and put some of the pieces of that night together, it does seem a challenge had been made. This night would precede my double cancer diagnoses by two years. Soon "the shape" of things would change. Was I being put to the test? Am I still?! Makes you wonder, doesn't it?

Chapter 6

EXPOSING A . . . mission?

So what do you think was the first thing the doctor was going to ask me to do?

Bingo! "Mr. Beck, I would like to begin with a physical exam, if that's okay?"

If you're a guy and have gone to see a urologist, you know there are really only two major things he's going to check. Of course, you tell the doctor it's okay to check. Why wouldn't it be okay? I don't know you, doc; we've never met, and you're another man. Sure. So, I act like it's no big deal. I think we do that so that we can tell ourselves, we're the one in control. Then there's the whole exposure thing. What is there to make of control? Of exposure? Or confidences, for that matter?

When it's been a while since you've been to the doctor, and it's just not your cup of tea, how's the whole process not supposed to be at least a little unnerving—especially if you're hiding your little secret? So, I stand there. I stand there like I'm not even in the room. I stand there eyes wide open seeing nothing. In time it was over and I would reenter my body, but not yet.

During this kind of exam the doctor will check your testicles and the prostate. Testicles are easy. Heck, they're kind of right out there. But the prostate, that's a different matter all together. The prostate gland is positioned just below your bladder, is about the size of a walnut, and your urinary canal runs smack dab through the middle of it. Funny thing: everything I have already told you should signal that it's located inside of your body! There's only one thing though. The prostate check is an internal external exam. There is a way to check the gland, but it's not pleasant. Let me introduce you to a friend to most men who have undergone this procedure. Say hello to "Mr. Jelly Finger"—otherwise known in urologist circles as the "urologist's handshake." I will spare you some of the other jokes, including one used regularly by a long time friend and doctor. Just picture those circus marvels who twirl plates on long slender sticks. You bend over the exam table, a little lubricant is applied, and up the index finger goes. And that's enough of that, Ta-Da. Men joke that you always want to pick your doctor by the size of his fingers—it's a coping mechanism really—but we all laugh, and move on.

The doctor would begin his physical exam with my testicles. The doctor, nurse, and I had been exchanging pleasantries about life and faith, as I often wear t-shirts that make some statement about my Christian faith, until he examined that left testicle. It stopped him in his tracks! I don't recall even getting to the second check of the prostate. I do recall him saying in a most animated way, "It's not that I'm not interested in your prostate, and I'm sure that will be fine anyway, but we need to get that testicle checked out right away!"

He wasn't joking. He had been standing with shoulders kind of rounded, casually. Now he stood at attention. His easy smile became a look like when you're caught in trouble. It wasn't a glare; it was an "I need your attention" kind of look. Eyes focused tightly right at me. He was at attention, and he wanted me to do likewise. Face, and shoulders forward, his voice was crisp and his tone strong and caring. His casual demeanor became one of great concern. He changed. The air in the room changed. No more fun and games. I had set the tone, all smiles, easy conversation about work and faith and life. This was no big deal even though I had known for two years that this was going to be a big deal. No more disassociation with what was going on. No more hiding the truth.

His orders went from "I'm sure this is going to be OK, but we'll give it a look," to "We need to get this checked out, and checked out right away! This has me concerned!"

Honestly, I was relieved. Having let you in on the secret already, I was glad that it was finally on the front burner. It would shape the days to come. I knew that too, but I just didn't know how. I remember telling the doctor just before I left, "I've got connections." Since we still needed to do something about my prostate number, the doctor scheduled a prostate biopsy to be done in his office, and I headed out the door.

As I walked across the parking lot the expressions I saw on his face and his words of urgency echoed in my head and flashed across my mind: "You need to get scheduled for an ultra sound of your testicle ASAP." This was one of those times when you usually hear, "I want it done yesterday!"

Evening came and went, and it was morning, the next day. I was back at my internship home away from home, Rush-Copley Hospital, the place I would go to offer help to the sick. There I was. Parking lots circle this large white complex. Doors leading in at various locations dot the exterior. Not unlike many of the hospitals you have visited, I suppose. Today it was my turn. I think it was about 10 AM, and this time there was no fancy shirt and tie or white chaplain's jacket; I was in street clothes. Once inside the building I headed for the outpatient area. This time I was the one waiting, watching, seated in one of those little clusters of chairs "for patients."

Rush-Copley's outpatient waiting room area was better lit than others I had visited. TVs positioned strategically provided something for our viewing pleasure. Except that most of the time I don't like the channel that's on and the volume is often a little louder than I would prefer. There's no escape. My ears strained, striving to hear what's of no interest to me. Thank the Lord I have become a reader. I position myself away from TVs and other patients, the loner corner. I wasn't there to make friends. I need it quiet when I read so I can concentrate—it's just the way I am.

Ironically, many who had seen me walk the halls in my chaplain coat found me sitting in the check in area. They weren't sure how to react; most were taken by surprise. I too was at a loss. This side is different than what I was used to. In time my name was called, "Mr. Beck." I yielded to the nurse and followed politely. They could be leading us anywhere, and I think we would follow.

A series of short hallways and doors later, I was in a small room with an examination table. "Please take a seat here on the exam table." The room was not cluttered with a lot of stuff. The walls were bare; I don't recall any chairs or desk of any kind, just the table and a portable ultrasound machine. Oh, and the room was not well lit. Actually, its lack of light seemed odd to me. I remember thinking that. So there I sat. In time a nice technician came in and introduced himself.

They always ask for your name. They just called me by it at least once already, but everyone has to ask. And your date of birth—let's not forget that, too. Once the formalities and introductions are over it's time to get down to the real reason for being there. "Mr. Beck, can I have you lower your pants and underwear for me and lay down on the table. Here's a towel." You do as they say. Inside I'm thinking, "Not again."

The test didn't scare me. But once more, exposure came to raise its ugly head. So I just began to turn stuff off. I did what was asked, and I heard the technician, but my mind disconnected me from what was happening around and to me. I listened as the technician gave me general instructions. He would use an ultrasound jelly with a small scanner like the instrument used to see a baby in a mother's womb. Baby ultrasounds are usually happy moments.

Soon it was clear. He showed me what my normal right testicle looked like, and then the abnormality of the left. Don't need to be a doctor for this one. Any one of us could have diagnosed the problem. I remember not having a lot of emotion. Remember, I had been living with this truth for two years. I had just finally gotten around to confirming it.

He took pictures, and said he would let the doctor know. He didn't make a diagnosis, of course, but it was clear. After all, a picture's worth a thousand words. Even I knew by what I saw.

I used the towel he had given me earlier to clean myself up. Up went the underpants, up went the shorts, zipped, buttoned, and belted. "Thanks," I said, and out the door I went. As usual, he informed me that the scans would be read and the findings sent to my doctor. "Have a nice day." I walked back through the waiting room, and out to my car. The sun was bright that day. Beautiful blue sky, temperature warm, warming, "Have a nice day" echoing in my head.

Back in my car I had one thing to do and one thing only: Call my wife. Liz knew why I was getting an ultrasound. So I made the call. She was at work. Can't say I recall just exactly what I said but I'm sure it sounded like many times before,

"It'll be okay. No big deal. Don't worry. They're just going to check some stuff out." I wonder if those words were for my benefit or hers?

STRANGE AND FAMILIAR

I think a lot of people have preconceived notions about what a calling is. Many of us attempt to live beyond ourselves, wanting to touch and be touched. I think of bands of young people scraping old paint off the side of an old building in parts of our own country foreign to them. I think of the Apostle Paul who made tents in between extended journeys to distant parts of his world.

By this time in my life I have learned what mission fields looked like for God and me. It's just a matter of watching, always being ready. I look with eyes that see beyond the human spectrum of vision. I know what to look for now. In between, moments pass as I perform the functions of my daily life. My mission fields are the places in which I live, the places where my heart beats. From my job to my run, from passing conversations that mysteriously present themselves, to organized meetings gathered around a table where we are fed by more than just the food, places and times serenely quiet or filled with noises as many gather around a common desire: each is a mission field. My life has seen many fields. Fields provide food; they can feed us if we let them.

My "field" work began when I heard a call from a voice that I didn't know and didn't recognize. Still, it filled the air I breathed. Whether during time with friends or moments spent in the tranquility of my own room, peace and purpose were born. I guess they had truly been birthed at my birth. In my infancy I didn't see what was staring me in the face. Soon, but still beyond my understanding, places of employment became fields readied before my opening eyes.

Co-workers, strangers on the street, people my wife and I would meet while on vacation, we would talk. They would come. I didn't have to look far. If you look closely, people are just dying to tell you their story. We all want to be known. We all want to be valued. We all want to be led to believe we have purpose and meaning. True, it's easy to be manipulative, but honesty stands the test of time. The human gut carries with it an immense amount of wisdom. Talk to someone, and it is not long before you know—you know inside—whether they are being honest and truthful.

By now I am sure you are beginning to draw some of your own conclusions about me, about my story. I am neither frightened you won't go on, nor scared that you won't believe me. I stand before you willing. I stand before those who know me—unashamed for who I am, and the blunt nature from which I often present my point of view.

I'm not sure of precisely when the Spirit spoke, that old familiar voice, but the message was clear. "Guy, this is a mission field." How simple. How clear the message came across my mind. I remember thinking, "Guy, you've witnessed in homes, at work, with friends and strangers, in bars, restaurant booths, and basements. But you've never witnessed in the medical arena." This was a call to speak to those who would be ministering to me.

It came to me as I walked across that parking lot that late afternoon. I know some of you are thinking, "Yeah, this was just a way he could give himself purpose so he could shift the attention off his ensuing cancer diagnosis." It's a free country. Think what you want. So here's what I think. Purpose is often driven by internal mechanisms, but calling finds its origins in the external and often divine.

My steps across that asphalt parking lot shifted from the steady pace of a metronome, to the uplifted stride of someone on a mission. I was excited for the opportunities, familiar and not, expectant with excitement at the mysterious prospects that would only be revealed in their time. My next field lay dead ahead—and I was all on board. It's easy to say now that this journey I'll call cancer would take many twists and turns. But as I told a friend once, "You know, a winding path never reveals its true length."

In synopsis, what can I say? Here we are together; we have walked through the winding path that has brought us to this parking lot today. While I know we are only getting started, that day brought a shift, a shift in perspective as I walked across yet another parking lot, leaving yet another doctor's office. It came like daylight to me from that darkened ultrasound exam room. It burst forth. I felt alive and back in the game. My heart beat faster; my eyes sharpened their focus; my mind raced with plans and strategies. Off the bench and into the game, joy like fireworks exploded onto the scene. This was a truly awesome day—every part of it.

Can you use *cancer* and *awesome* in the same sentence?

Chapter 7

Let the GAMES Begin

Peek-a-boo Pincushion

My mom still has this knitted pincushion that started as a strip of knitted yarn and then was rolled into a circular object about two to three inches in diameter. Funny, I never ever thought one day I would become one. Would anyone?

Guys, if you're squeamish, skip this section. This starts out real messy and ends up a real pain in the butt. I'm not sure I would have wanted to know this going in. (Get it— going in?) Anyway, here we are. I will tell this next part in the present as if it is happening—again. Not that I need to relive it, but maybe it will seem more real.

I took a day off work today. I used a sick day. One of those times though you would have rather been at work. And don't get me wrong: I'm not a workaholic. I like being off, but not so much today.

The morning begins with phase one of the mission, a trip to the grocery store pharmacy section. I need to pick up a Fleet enema. Sounds good already doesn't it? Today is the day when I have my prostate biopsied. So, first things first: you are told not to eat for at least twelve hours before because they need your system cleared out. And just to be sure, you are to give yourself a Fleet enema, which, let me tell you if you haven't had the pleasure, guarantees there is nothing left in any of that part of your system at all!

For those more experienced at this art I apologize for my lack of grace in completing this required task. I wonder: do I look like a yoga instructor or some kind of body contortionist? In high school I competed in gymnastics. My event was the still rings, so I've stood on my head a lot. I've also made my body do all kinds of unusual things in the name of stretching in order to perform my still rings routines, but none of those things prepared me for this. I'm sorry, but trying to make sure I got all the contents of that bottle of liquid exactly where it belonged was no simple task. What a nightmare! I found it to be rather humiliating, even if no one was watching.

"Phewwww." I'm glad that was over with, but now the clock starts ticking. Like in the movies, someone starts the timer on a bomb and we all start counting down, and waiting, and counting, watching for the explosion. I wasn't going far, just in case. A bomb is ticking inside me, just waiting to go off. Unlike in the movies, no one came in to save the day. All I'm going to say is, boy did it go off! I was really glad that was over. I recall calling my wife who was at work to ask for some pointers, but thankfully she didn't have any more experience with this than I did. I should have called someone who was a veteran with these things, but who wants to tell anyone they are the "go to" person when it comes to using Fleet enemas? I wouldn't let that get out, if I could help it. Finally, sparing you any further nasty details, that was that, mission accomplished!

So here we go, ANOTHER drive to the doctor's office. I thought to describe my drive past local landmarks, traffic signals, and the maze of traffic that goes with suburban living, but then I don't suppose my drive is much different than yours. Close your eyes and I'll bet at least some of you know the way by heart. The doctor's office used to be a building I just drove by. It carried with it no internal or external significance. Boy, times change, and so do locations we remember, don't they? It's not exactly like highlight locations from a family trip. We don't take keepsake snapshots of our nice smiling faces or hit the gift shop on the way out, do we? How ironic that familiar landmarks carry with them attached meanings when you think about it.

Oh, here we are! I almost drive right by. Sometimes, OK, most times, my friends say I talk too much. But we were having such a nice philosophical conversation. I like running stuff like that around in my brain. I find it very interesting and enjoy opportunities to sit and talk over such things. Well, I guess I'd better park the car rather than keep talking. Don't want to be late for my appointment, you know.

We'll skip the waiting room stuff. You've been there twice already. I'm sure you almost know it as well as I by now. Sorry, just the way it is.

The usual nurse's hale, "Mr. Beck." Up I bounce, nice smile, warm hello—at least I hope it was. A day full of promise. I followed the female assistant. She didn't know me as well then as she soon would. I'm sorry for that too. As I walk in I notice a metal tray on a small rolling cart about the size of a normal TV tray. The kind most of us have in our homes. My eyes quickly do the math. Twelve. There were twelve little swatches or small squares on the tray. The nurse had covered the tray with a larger towel, but done a poor job. My guess is they wanted to keep the twelve as a surprise. Failed!

She asks me to sit over on the exam table and offers some small talk. Twelve. That was the number. She goes on with some more small talk, and so do I. Twelve. That's the image burned into your mind. More blah-blah-blah. Twelve. I just couldn't get that number out of my head. In time she begins with some of the medical stuff. It's time to cut to the chase. I say, "Let me just stop you there and tell you that whatever you're going to do to me, I already know you're going to do it TWELVE times."

"Oh, you noticed the tray!" she says.

I really wanted to yell, "Which did you think I am, dumb or blind?" But I don't. Instead, I opt for, "Well, it's pretty obvious when you have a shiny stainless steel tray with twelve little swatches of stuff on it, and I'm here for a tissue biopsy of my prostate. It's not hard to figure out." So we got that out of the way. The only thing we are waiting on now is the doctor.

In time, he comes in. Phase four—the biopsy. Time to hear those nice explanations of what they're going to do to you. I know I have already told you how they locate the prostate gland. Do I need to remind you again?

So they want to take twelve tissue samples from a gland located out of sight only approachable through your rectum. It's kind of like a puzzle. So how do they do that? I know you're all dying to know. They use some sort of an ultrasound device that I can't describe because the good Lord put our eyes on the opposite side of our bodies, and I have never wanted to look it up on the Internet or ask my doctor to show me.

It was truly one of the most uncomfortable feelings I had ever experienced. Probing with the ultrasound thing, watching on their monitor, it's kind of like real estate: location,

location, location. In the end (ha-ha) I'm not sure how the doctor decides where and when to pull the trigger, but it still boils down to dividing up a walnut twelve ways.

The moment of truth arrives. The doctor asks me to lie on the table on my left side. Once more my pants are at my knees. There we are, all three of us. I must say the discomfort is very discomforting. Just getting the probe in is no fun at all. Then the doctor begins to move it around and, BAM! He fires off his gizmo sending a needle through the wall of my rectum and into the prostate gland grabbing a small piece of tissue. When satisfied with shot number one, the doctor moves it around once more preparing to fire again. I audibly groan, unsettled, unnerved, humiliated, and BAM! He lets it rip again. Two down, ten to go. I just want it to be over, and over quickly. Ouch, maybe "rip" was the wrong choice of words. Lest I be painfully redundant, I won't say "reposition, BAM," anymore.

In time twelve samples are gathered from twelve different locations, top to bottom, side to side, and middle. The by-product is some rectal bleeding. They tell me I should watch that. Blood from your rectum—when does that ever sound good? They also give me an antibiotic, just in case, for all the puncture wounds, a precaution so you don't get an infection from the procedure. I am also told to pay attention to the color of the blood. Bright red blood would mean continued fresh bleeding. Darker blood is old, clotted blood. They say that some bleeding could continue for a few days. Just one more thing to keep an eye on. Oh, boy.

Now for the drive home. No, I don't care that there is still some discomfort following me out the door. I am just glad to get out of there. Residual pain is to be expected. I'm racking my brain now, and for the life of me I don't remember if they gave me a pad or something for inside my underwear. I do remember that the post-puncture bleeding went on for a few hours. That I recall.

You know, by now I'm not waxing quite so philosophical. I appreciate your coming along; it helped. I think on the ride home we'll just listen to some music or sit quietly, if you don't mind. Thanks for understanding.

DAILY DOUBLE

Now, I'm not necessarily a fan of the Jeopardy TV show; most times it makes me feel like an idiot, or confirms that I am. But there are those moments in the show when the cube-shaped answer reveals those two special words, "Daily Double." The bells sound, the contestant's heart beats a little faster. Everyone sits on the edges of their seats. This could really make or break a contestant's chances of winning. A silence falls over the suspended seconds like the hush of an audience when the house lights dim. Everybody listens, watching for any hint given by the contestant that he or she knows the right question or not. The moment is ripe for victory or defeat. Hit it, and you're a big winner. Everyone loves winners. Then the contestant says, "What is . . .?"

That's how it felt as I arrived for my third visit to the initial urologist who did my physical exam and biopsy of the prostate. We meet again. Same office, same nice staff, same, same, same. This meeting was to discuss the results of the prostate biopsy and the ultrasound of my left testicle.

You know the drill. Everyone's friendly. The doctor walks in and sits down, my results in hand, hidden away in one of those mysterious folders that hold the keys to your life. I've never seen inside one of those folders. I wonder if I held my doctor's file—his life—in my hand, might he look at these folders differently?

It wasn't long. Of course, I just sat there. It's not like I came for a game of cards or something. "Well, Mr. Beck I received the results from your biopsy and I regret to inform you that the biopsy found cancerous cells in your prostate." Then they gave me my Gleason score.

A Gleason score is the sum total of two numbers, the primary and secondary degradation of what is considered normal cells found when viewed under a microscope. Primary identifies the cells of the most deformation and location. The secondary number identifies the condition of the cells in what is determined to be the secondary location of concern. I understand them to be similar to severity and speed—how bad the worse spot is and how fast the secondary spot will look as bad as the worse spot.

I'm not a doctor, so if you want the doctor's definition, ask one, or check with your computer under Gleason score info and get the scoop for yourself. I was a 6, 3 + 3.

Oh, one more thing. The doctor also had the pathology results on the testicle as well. Ding, ding, ding—it's the Daily Double. "Mr. Beck, I'm sorry to inform you that your testicle was found to be cancerous as well—seminoma, malignant tumor of the testicle."

"OK," is all I could manage to say. It's not like I didn't think the testicle was cancerous. Admittedly, the prostate surprised me, but what's a guy to do? I knew the PSA number was also suspicious. He admitted that this was not normal at all.

I remember his words, "You're too old for the one, and too young for the other. We really don't see people your age with these combinations of cancers."

I like being an over-achiever. Having had conversations with the doctor about my faith in the past, I told him, "I've got connections, if you know what I mean." And that's all there is to that.

The doctor proceeded to tell me that surgery for the testicle was the normal course of action, and that made perfect sense. But the prostate is a different matter altogether. Let's review some of the options. This isn't Prostate 101, and it's not going to be overly scientific, but here are some of your choices. You can have surgery to remove the prostate gland entirely, have radioactive seeds placed in the prostate to kill the cells in the affected areas, have proton beam therapy which kind of does the same thing but with a beam, or general radiation. The list changes as our technology changes.

Options depend on the person's age, general health, and personal preference. Sometimes older patients are advised not to do anything at all, because the cancer can be slow growing. You may be old enough where it will not matter in the end.

So much for generalizations. At that moment, I was the guy. The doctor looked at me and said, "Mr. Beck, because you're only 47, it would be my recommendation that you have both your testicle and prostate removed surgically. I would be glad to do the surgeries, but I would like to recommend that you contact a very good doctor at Loyola. Doctors who have prostate trouble call him. He's the doctor who writes the articles and teaches the techniques that the rest of the doctors are learning and using."

He sounded awesome.

My doctor continued, "He's the best of the best, but, . . ."

" But what?" I asked.

" Well, he's very difficult to see. He is in high demand, but you could try giving him a call. Your case is out of the norm, so maybe he will see you."

"I told you—remember Doc—I've got connections. If it's supposed to be, it will happen." I thanked the doctor for all he had done, and told him I'd let him know.

I left the office with three things: testicular cancer, prostate cancer, and a small piece of paper. The paper with a very short list of who's who in Urology had one number on it— I was appealing my case straight to the top.

I walked across the parking lot once more, and opened the door to my car. It was about 4:30 in the afternoon. I got in the car and dialed the number right from the parking lot.

I was thinking: it's only 4:30. Most doctors' offices stay open till at least five; it's worth a shot, rather than waiting until tomorrow.

A voice answers. "Hello. This is Dr. Frank's office. My name is Robin. Can I help you?"

CONNECTIONS
OF THE INVISIBLE KIND

"Can I help you?" What an odd question to ask someone who is calling a doctor's office. You know, sometimes when you call someone for the first time you just don't know how to begin, especially when it's important. This was one of those times. So, I kind of jump right in. "Well, my name is Mr. Beck and I was given Dr. Frank's name, because I was just diagnosed with both testicular and prostate cancer. The doctor I just saw said my case is unusual and suggested I give Dr. Frank a call, and just maybe he would see me."

"So let me get this straight," she said. "You were given Dr. Frank's name by referral?"

"Yes."

"So why again were you told to call Dr. Frank?"

"Well, my doctor said that Dr. Frank is the leader in his field. He said he's the guy the doctors go to if they need a doctor. I'm 47 years old and have just been diagnosed with both testicular and prostate cancer. The other doctor said I'm too old for one and too young for the other, and I have them both. He said maybe Dr. Frank would see me."

I heard nothing. Pause. Dead air, almost to the point where I wanted to say "Hello" again to see if we were still connected. Then Robin came back on the phone, "Can you come tomorrow at five o'clock? He will be working out of the Oak Brook office. Would you be able to make it for five?"

"ABSOLUTELY!" I think was my response. If not, insert

66

any word you might use to let the other person know that come hell or high water there is nothing that could stand in your way. I had been told it could take a long time, if he would consider my case at all. "TOMORROW, at five I'll be there," and hung up the phone! I like the word "absolutely." It leaves no room for ambiguity. There's not much in life that seems absolute any more, but this was.

Once home I told Liz about the appointment and Dr. Frank and his reputation. I told her I was going to see him in Oakbrook Terrace at five tomorrow. Liz informed me that "WE" would be seeing him at five.

The next morning, the first thing I did was to check when my urologist's office would be open. I needed my records, and fast. It's kind of an oxymoron to speak about doctors' offices and fast in the same sentence. Once I knew the time, I kept checking my watch every minute or so. When the time finally came I made the call.

When the receptionist answered, I told her my name and mentioned the doctor who had referred me to Dr. Frank, and since I would be seeing Dr. Frank today at five, they needed to send my records over to his Oak Brook office. She asked when I last spoke to my urologist. I told her, " Yesterday afternoon. That's when she said I should give Dr. Frank a call."

"And you're seeing him WHEN?"

"Today at five."

Silence. She asked me if I could please hold. The next voice I heard was that of my urologist. "My receptionist said you're asking to have your records transferred."

"Yep, to Dr. Frank's Oak Brook office. You said I should call him, so I did last night when I left your office."

"And you're seeing him today at five?" It was more a question then a statement. "YES." More silence.

"Nobody sees him that fast!"

"Well, I am! And I need my records there by five." Even more silence, and then before he could speak, I said,

"Remember Doc, I told you I have connections." That was the last time I ever spoke to him.

Liz and I met up back up at home late that afternoon. We gathered our things and jumped in the car heading for Oak Brook. It took about 30 minutes to get there. Another brick office building. We found the entrance and walked in. It seemed like they were closing shop for the day. I got the impression I was the last person to be seen. We went through all the usual photocopying of insurance cards and ID and stuff. I was handed the typical clipboard full of questions about health history, name, address, phone; every office has them. It is what they do. It is what we do as patients. So, I filled it out. Then we waited.

Soon a nurse called my name, so we followed her down the hall to a small exam room on the left. It was painted white. A small desk and two chairs were on the left as you entered. It had the usual exam table with the long strip of paper stretched out along its length. The walls were adorned with little art work. I've come to notice how some offices use art more than others. I think it is supposed to soothe us. Of course, right alongside the art are those anatomical posters of male organs. It is a urology office, after all. The walls also had one of those photocopied sheets of paper with simple faces showing different expressions. You know, the faces they use to determine pain levels. Odd combinations when you think about it. Like the painting is supposed to make my eyes invisible to all of the other stuff that reminds me I am not here just to relax and enjoy the painting!

As I sat down, the nurse asked me about my health history and the reason for the visit. So I gave her the "too young—too old" speech. She took some more notes. Then she began to leave the room, but then turned, half in the room and half out. "You know Dr. Frank is the best. Not just anybody gets to see Dr. Frank." Then she left. Liz and I looked at each other, eye to eye. Without speaking, Liz and I both thought,

"That was odd." It was abrupt, and she was clearly making a point for our benefit.

Soon a tall distinguished gentleman walked in the room and extended his hand, "I'm Dr. Frank. I half stood up, shook his hand, and introduced myself and my wife. He was not pretentious. He had a calm and friendly demeanor, and we chatted some. You know how your gut knows. My gut was telling me, he's the guy. He's STILL the guy.

As you can figure, he too wanted to do a physical check, so Liz left the room. Once again the tube of KY jelly and rubber gloves came out. Wham-bam-slam—here we go again. Little did I know how many times that was going to happen in my future. With that done and my testicle checked, Liz came back into the room. He explained the course of action he would recommend. "First, we are going to do the removal of the testicle." He didn't care if he or my original doctor did that surgery, and said so. He said that surgery needed to be done at the first possible opportunity. Six weeks later, he said "he" would do the second surgery on the prostate. He is the man. The recovery from the prostate surgery would also be six weeks following a brief hospital stay.

Dr. Frank asked if we understood, and if we were OK with the plan. We said we understood and thought it sounded good. "Sounded good?" Wow. We shook hands once more and we headed home. I don't think we were in his exam room for fifteen minutes. The whole visit was maybe thirty tops, if you count from the time we walked in, and the next three to four months of our lives had just been mapped out. WE never saw this as part of any future Liz or I dreamt of.

The next morning I would call the urologist who had made the referral to schedule the date for the testicular surgery. It would be performed by a colleague of his. He was going to be out of the office.

So you know what that meant. I would need to schedule another appointment with his colleague, because he, too, insisted on seeing me before he would do the surgery. That appointment was straightforward. It also took place in one of those nondescript exam rooms. He also wanted to do a physical exam of the testicle he would be removing. Why not, I thought. Everyone else has. I went alone for that visit. It was brief.

Come to think of it, I think I saw three different doctors over the course of about one week. I think the surgery was scheduled to happen in a week or a little more. I left his office with another hurdle complete, one last hurdle to go before the first big show.

IT'S AN ACQUIRED TASTE

Maybe what it really needs is one of those little umbrellas—dress it up a little. Yea, that'll do the trick. In the short window of time just prior to the surgery to remove my left testicle, I stood at the kitchen counter with a small bottle of this milky whitish liquid. I was to add this bottle to water to make four full cups of liquid.

I was to drink the milky, slimy liquid two cups at a time. The first two cups were very difficult. It didn't go down easy, and I can think of a lot better things to drink than four cups of this stuff. Two cups at bedtime, two cups as soon as I wake up. Those were the orders that came with the bottle.

Awaking to test day, the second two cups of barium sat perched on the shelf in the fridge. "What's for breakfast, Honey?" Who are you kidding? I took the cold barium off the shelf and poured it into a container that would hold all of the remaining two cups. I could feel my pulse increase, and anxiety level rise as well. I took a few deep breaths, closed my eyes, "DOWN THE HATCH," I thought in my head. Wow. For me it comes off as slimy in consistency, making it hard to swallow. Still, I just kept swallowing until the cup was empty. I was glad when it was over once and for all.

Liz and I drove to Copley and parked the car. It was the day of my first CAT scan. We waited patiently in the waiting room. In my mind, I can still see where we sat. As you walked in there was a counter to your left where you were welcomed by the admissions person. They would politely ask you your name. Then they would ask you to take a seat.

The admissions counter was followed by a much longer counter area that was divided into cubicles. Here records and insurance persons in turn would call your name, go over your personal information and double check your appointment status. Then you would sit down in the waiting room and wait for your name to be called.

In a short time, a woman appeared with a wax paper cup. She called my name, and I answered. "Mr. Beck, we need you to drink this." She handed me the cup then she walked away. More barium to drink, but this time it was pink. They had added some sweetened drink mixture to it to change the flavor. I stared into the cup. They may have changed the flavor and color, but it didn't change the consistency. I can still see the cup right now. I looked at it; I looked at Liz. I opened my mouth to drink but only managed about two small swallows. I felt flushed, and began to perspire. I looked at Liz. She looked at me and asked if I was OK. We both knew I was anything but OK.

All I remember saying was, "You know, if I drink one more swallow of this stuff, it's all coming right back up. I just can't get down another swallow." Quietly, Liz took the cup from my hand without a word and walked it over to the counter and informed them it just wasn't going to happen. They seemed to understand. Maybe, just maybe, I wasn't the first to react this way.

Soon it came time for the testing. As testing goes, this is the easy part. I entered another small room where another medical person inserted an IV into my arm. Being my first time through all this I had no idea what that was for. But again, you go along. They ran my scan test with and without contrast. So what does that mean? It means they scan your body twice. Oh, and just before you lie on the scanner table they ask you to drink another small cup of barium.

Anyway, "without contrast" is a scan of your body with barium only, and that's done first. "With contrast" means adding an injection of iodine into your body through an IV line they insert as part of the prep for the scans. The iodine coursing through your veins somehow highlights your organs and stuff differently than when it is done without the iodine. When they add the iodine it comes with a reminder, or warning, from the radiologist. The injection of iodine creates a metallic taste in your mouth and makes you feel warm and fuzzy—but only in your lower regions, as if you just peed in your pants.

The test is done as you lie on the table. The table is then moved forward and backward through a large ring that encircles the table. At times, while they are scanning you, you are directed to breathe. It is a somewhat mechanical voice coming from the scanner, "Breathe in, hold your breath." You move back and forth, "Breathe." There are also little faces on the scanner, one face looks like someone holding his breath with cheeks puffed out. The other, you guessed it, is a face that has exhaled with lines that show breath moving out from your mouth. All the while your body is somehow radiated in a way that lets them see you internally. Cross sections are taken of your body, in my case in three millimeter increments. I just learned that at my last visit. I had never asked before. They scan my chest, abdomen, and pelvis.

The scan from start to finish took no more than 30 minutes. Honestly, I don't remember much of that first scan. I don't remember how it went, or even how I got out of there. I don't even remember the drive home. My brain isn't interested in remembering that, I guess.

Over the past six years I don't know how many gallons of barium I have been asked to drink. The first was by far the worst. Over time it has gotten to be no big deal. I prefer my barium at room temperature, thank you very much. When it's cold, your stomach doesn't let you get it down as fast. By now I don't mind the flavor, even though it's not great. I drink it straight up. I don't mind the consistency either, any more. I can shoot two cups of barium in no time. If it's warm I can take a deep breath and chug the whole thing like a machine. Just keep swallowing. I don't like looking into the cup. You just stare off, like when you're looking out into space but not seeing. I don't add flavor, never did. Like I said, I like my barium straight up.

I don't relish the experience. It's just the way it is. We can choose to make the best of it or not. Each time I get my bottle now, I like to make some kind of joke with the woman behind the counter. That's where I first suggested she dress it up with a small umbrella, like one of those beach drinks. The last time she smiled and laughed. She acknowledged how nasty it tastes and questioned why the flavor had not been improved. If you are out there—you barium creators—please see what you can do about the flavor and consistency, could you? It would really be appreciated, thanks.

As of late, news channels around by us have covered hospital stories in which patients had received doses of radiation well beyond the recommended dose in the course of their CT scans. Some days it makes me wonder. Will all the radiation be the cause of some other form of cancer I didn't already have? Or, what about drinking all that barium and being injected with iodine? They assure us this stuff is safe, don't they? I don't give much brain time to worrying about this, but I can't say it hasn't crossed my mind.

GREGG'S GIFT

Gregg's gift was really not all that unusual as gifts go. It was his way of saying, "Get well." The gift is a blue-gray t-shirt, size medium, standard crew neck with short sleeves. On the front is a cartoon drawing of a tree with three squirrels perched on one of its lower limbs, each clutching a nut except for one squirrel.

The day of my first surgery arrived. As many of you know, you are asked to arrive many hours before the scheduled time. Day surgery, yes, that's the place. I arrived with Liz early that morning. It was your typical August day in the Midwest. The morning sun was bright; the day would be warm, but not un-bearably hot. Liz dropped me off at the door I think, and then parked the car.

We walked in together, Liz carrying her supplies and mine. Supplies included a newspaper, some books, and an as-sortment of small things she might try to do while waiting. Waiting rooms are called that for a reason. With all the other souls—you wait. I wasn't nervous. Look, it had to be done; that's all there is to that. Actually, I was relieved. This had been hanging over my head for two years. Finally having it taken care of was a relief. I had been afraid before—before when I knew and did nothing. So as days go, this was a good day! Besides, I had never had surgery or been under general anesthetic before. So what's to worry about? I felt a level of ex-citement inside. The whole thing felt more like an adventure rather than a surgery. It was kind of cool.

At Copley they had nice little day rooms set up. This meant Liz could spend more of the time with me, at least until it was my turn. As per instructions I removed all of my clothes and put on one of those very stylish hospital gowns, size who knows. Let's just say there was more than enough fabric for my needs; I'm 5'6" tall and weigh 135 lbs.

We waited. Liz sat in a chair by the window, and I was supposed to lie in the bed, again per instructions. Every so often a nice nurse would appear and let us know how much longer it might be. I think the TV was on, or we read. Those of you who are finding this vaguely familiar, have you ever been given a time for your surgery and found it to be accurate? Like a bear readying itself for hibernation we hunkered down for a long winter's nap.

Finally, it was my turn. They brought in a gurney and asked me to lie on it. "No problem." I told them. I hopped on it like kids at a carnival when it's their turn on the ride. Down the hall we rolled—a very nondescript hall at that with muted colors on the walls and rather plain linoleum on the floor. It was like one of a thousand similar halls. Who cares? I was being wheeled on the gurney by two male nurses, or techs, or some combo, I'm not exactly sure. They were two guys; let's leave it at that. They made some small talk amongst themselves first, and then with me. We knew where I was headed—surgery. And, I'm sure they probably knew what for. Then it dawned on me.

So, I looked up at the two guys and said, "Look at it this way guys, at least when I come out I'll be half as nuts as when I went in." I smiled. They looked shocked. "Did you hear what he just said?" one asked the other. He nodded in the affirmative and pushed open the door on the operating room. They never said another word. Those guys needed to loosen up. Come on. That was funny. At least that's the way I saw it.

Once inside the operating room the orderlies positioned me next to the operating table. The OR table was surrounded by what seemed to be an assortment of staff—anesthesiologist, nurses, etcetera, but no surgeon as of yet. I think it was the nurse who asked me if I would slide over onto the operating table. "Piece of cake," I said, and over I slid. Standing directly behind my head was a pleasant-looking man. The large round lights of the OR encircled the table poised for action.

Oh, one thing I do remember very well was the warm blankets they put on you. The room was cold, but the blankets were awesome. They might not have needed to put me out. Those warm blankets would have done the trick if they'd let them. Nap time was coming.

Soon the man standing behind my head asked me how I was feeling. Never having gone under general anesthesia before, I told him things were looking fuzzy. I felt as fuzzy as things looked. It was the weirdest thing. I never saw the shot administered into my IV, but that didn't matter. Someone slipped me a Mickey, and I knew exactly who it was: the man standing right behind me. He mentioned that soon I would be out and asked me to count backwards from 100. I think I got to 96; I don't remember anything after that. Lights out, I slept like a baby.

I remember nothing of the surgery, of course, but, via my brother, I was told that when the nurse kept trying to check my BP I would pull my arm away from her and growl. In time I awoke from la-la land, back in bed, back in that nice day surgery room. Liz was there and asked how I was feeling. I felt great. I am sure the drugs played a role in that. So, there I was, dressed in my fashionable hospital gown a stylish new jock strap to keep things in order, and pretty brown hospital socks. You know, the ones with the fancy tread patterns on the bottom. There I lay, all smiles.

The nurse had given Liz my discharge orders: no lifting more than eight pounds, no running, and no walking for a while either. I was to get lots of rest, and no going to work for four to six weeks. Liz read, I slept some more.

Eventually the drugs had run their course and I was ready for discharge. It was then that Chaplain Dan arrived. You remember, head chaplain for the hospital. He commented that I looked great and offered me a ride out in a wheelchair. I was standing by the counter as Liz took care of some last-minute paperwork. I still don't know if it was policy that you had to be wheeled out. I told Dan, "I walked in on my own two legs, and I'm walking out on my own two legs." Liz looked at Dan, Dan looked at Liz, and I said, "Let's go!" and headed out the door with everything but a left testicle. My left testicle headed off to the lab.

Here's a little piece of general information. When something abnormal is identified in one or both of your testicles they don't biopsy, because they don't want to risk a wayward cell getting away. They just remove the whole testicle along with some of the connective parts. The goal is complete removal, and no escapees.

For those of you who are more curious then most, to remove your testicle they make an incision in your groin about two inches long to the right or left of center depending upon which testicle is being removed. They also used stitches rather than staples. In some cases the doctor can add an artificial testicle. I wasn't given the option. I wasn't asked.

The pathologists and the lab personnel all knew me and knew I was having this surgery, so everyone gathered around the specimen like kids at a campfire. The only thing left was to section, freeze the sample, make shavings, and identify what is going on under the microscope.

At home I sat on the couch watching TV. I have no idea what was on, but if you were to ask me, I was fine, perfectly fine. Liz kept checking with me, and the phone kept ringing. It's nice to have friends who care. I answered one call from Jason, a work friend. Quickly Liz grabbed the phone out of my hand. I was speaking absolute gibberish, I guess. She laughed and assured them I was OK.

They prescribed Vicodin for pain management once home. Vicodin makes me sleepy and nothing more. I used Vicodin for the remainder of that day, and then switched to generic pain meds. I would rather suffer through some pain than ever run the risk of pain meds that have addictive properties. It felt great to be home. Home should feel great.

Oh, I almost forgot to tell you what the t-shirt said. I'm sure you remember how the cartoon showed three squirrels perched on a lower limb of a tree. Each squirrel holding a nut except for one squirrel. That one was looking down in a very sad, forlorn sort of a way as he watched his nut falling to the ground. The caption read, "It's all fun and games until some-one loses a nut."

When I first began wearing the t-shirt to work you should have seen some of the looks I got, or even comments. I guess they didn't expect me to be able to laugh at what was obvi-ously a pretty good joke. I've been wearing it now for six years, I wore it again just the other day, and it is still getting laughs. Even Gregg and I still share a good chuckle. By now the color has faded, and the neckline is tattered from wear. I didn't keep it hidden in the drawer. That would have been no way to treat a gift from the heart of a friend.

COME TO THINK OF IT

Does anyone really go looking for this kind of stuff? I didn't. But my mind kept mulling all the effects of this stuff over and over. Both a blessing and a curse, wanted and yet unwanted, I began to use its effects to harden my resolve and reshape my thoughts.

If I may ask, any of you out there reading this who have had cancer: did you go looking for it? For the vast major-ity of us, cancer doesn't strike because of something we did or didn't do. Still, it's likely you want to blame yourself. Of course, you may be one of those persons doing something that we all know is a huge contributor to cancer. Smoking fits in that category. We've all heard the warnings—and still some of us choose to ignore them. All I can say is, "Maybe you shouldn't be surprised if or when it happens." Hopefully you may still have enough time to dig in your heels and take the steps you need to take before it is too late.

I shouldn't have to tell you. I'm sure you know who you are. Family members shouldn't have to tell you either, or beg, as the case may be. You know the only reason they keep try-ing to tell you is because they love you. Maybe if you don't care about yourself, you should do it for them. What message are you sending them if you don't change the necessary behavior?—Hmm . . . I'll leave that right there.

Most of us don't go looking for cancer. So why do many seem to blame themselves or act like they should be ashamed? The honest truth is that nearly everyone at some time or another has had something happen to them that they never went looking for. But while it still remains true that most of us don't go looking for events like a cancer diagnosis, there seems to be an interesting shift in the social fabric when it happens.

During these years following my surgeries the social climate concerning cancer seems to be radically changing. What I am finding most interesting is the subculture being created by cancer. Society has been creating these subcultures for a long time: "While he was in Bethany in the home of a man known as *Simon the Leper...*" (italics added for emphasis). Amazingly, this quote comes to us from around AD 30.

Did you know, back in those days lepers were often separated from society, FORCED to live in separate colonies away from "normal" society? Did you know that every time someone came near you, if you were a leper, you were required to yell out, "LEPER! LEPER!" How'd you like that? This really began to come into focus for me as my situation unfolded. What if you and I were required by society to shout out the diseases we have, or have had?

Now, I'm not stupid. I know that some things were done in the past out of ignorance. I also know that people with certain afflictions needed to be separated to decrease the possibility of contagion. I am also well aware of the fact that these people were often ostracized, due to no fault of their own.

News flash! Aren't we doing the same thing to ourselves today? Isn't society segmenting us from "normal" society every day? Aren't many cancer patients willingly creating these same subcultures? There seems to have developed a misguided, though well-meaning, social structure that highlights cancer patients unlike any other known disease. Why? I can think of many less "popular" diseases that can be a lot worse to die from than cancer. Don't many of us in our own way call out "CANCER, CANCER!" everywhere we go, willingly identifying ourselves daily?

What I want is someone to explain to me why? This "why" just kept gnawing at me as people tried to label me. It seemed all I kept hearing was, "My cancer this . . . ," "My cancer that. . . ." I couldn't shake the "why." Why were so many people treating themselves this way? Why? Isn't it just a disease?

Every time I felt bombarded by this pressure I can remember telling myself, "You can keep it!" I hated the way it just kept gnawing at me. I hated it. What I hated more was the hold I felt it had on others, but I never spoke up. I watched and watched, growling inside, letting it fester like an infected wound. If there was any real form of a cancer inside of me, this was it. This cancer I hated. Over and over I kept reciting the words, "Do we really want to make it ours? Do we?" My jaw would clench, my fists would clench, my gut would clench. I needed a cure. We're fighting for the cure, aren't we?

I thought, there are twenty eight million of us, and the vastness of that number too consumed my thinking. I thought about this more than what was next on my schedules with hospitals, doctors, or tests, or surgeries. Each time I would have to go again to the hospital, doctor, or for tests, this wound was opened up all over again as I watched the numberless faces, you and me, all twenty eight million of us. I just kept thinking twenty-eight million seemed like a pretty powerful group for a revolt. The embers of REVOLT began to burn hotter and hotter.

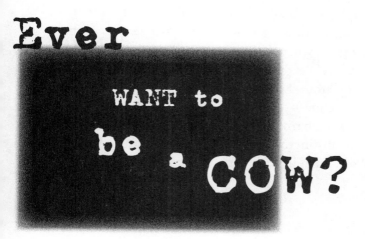

Chapter 8

Ever WANT to be a COW?

Ever give cows much thought?

I have for some dumb reason. We travel the country roads of Wisconsin. One day I noticed that besides corn, you see a lot of cows. Herds and herds of cows. Most of the cows I have seen are Holsteins, I think. But, since I am not a cow identification expert we'll just identify them as the black and white ones. They all look the same.

Often, and for reasons yet unexplainable to me, I have wondered, even aloud. "Is there anything going on inside a cow's head? Do they think? What do they do all day, standing in various groups by the barn, or as they lie in an adjacent pasture?" I know this may seem odd to you, but I've wondered.

It's funny to me. They rise to a new day. Do they know it's a new day? A day bright with sunshine, knee deep in mud, you know, in that one big mud puddle that seems common to every farmyard where cows are kept. They just stand knee deep in mud—NO expression—just stand there while the sun shines brightly around them.

Then somehow—another mystery to me—they start that march to the barn, every morning, every late afternoon. Someone, one instinctively knows it's her turn to go first, and the rest follow. Each in their turn, they march to the barn.

Chapter 9

Perceptions

Do I look like Humpty Dumpty to you?

Others react to those of us with cancer in lots of different ways. Those reactions are as diverse as the types of cancer one can have. Not everyone may want you to overcome your cancer, believe it or not. Some may be hoping to see you crash and burn. While that may sound absolutely crazy, it can be true regardless of how it sounds.

During my recovery from my first surgery, I encountered a variety of reactions—shock, surprise, concern, bewilderment, and disbelief. What I didn't realize was that there are those who are silently watching. They are watchers who have their own feelings about your fight with cancer—especially if you're a Christian. Christian? Why should that matter? It matters, because they want to see you crack. They want to see your faith fail you. They want to see you question God in a way that will validate their right to disbelieve.

At work, I am both liked and disliked, as is probably true of most of us. There are those I am closer to, those I only have the most informal contact with, and many in between. At work I can be outspoken about my opinions and faith; it's part of who I am.

My faith is something that became very personal to me back in 1976. I was nineteen when my neighbor friend Eric witnessed to both my brother and me. That's the night that it all made sense to me. That night I made "my own" personal decision about the validity of who Jesus was as my Savior. Let's just say that I have been pretty outspoken about my faith to others ever since.

This includes where I work. Work is no different. Throughout my varying jobs and places of employment, many have sought me out to ask questions, discuss difficulties, seek guidance during life struggles, or just argue about why my beliefs are wrong or misguided. My openness about what I believe has helped others find it easy to talk with me, whether we agree or not.

But there are others who do not appreciate your freedom of faith. Instead, they choose to make fun of your faith, and God, or Jesus. They would rather crack jokes. It is people like this who are out there hoping to see you fall. Sometimes we know who they are; sometimes we don't.

"Humpty Dumpty sat on a wall, Humpty Dumpty had a great fall" goes the nursery rhyme. It was during the early days following my two diagnoses and first surgery that I began to get a sense that something was growing inside me, but it wasn't cancer.

My attitudes and thinking about life, faith, and cancer were changing. Growing within me were the first revisions of my thinking about life and faith that I will discuss more fully later. It was in the course of these internal changes that an invisible force was challenging my faith. What I didn't know was that some who were watching were quietly hoping I would fail. That my faith would fail. It was in this climate that a friend came to me saying, "You know they're watching you. They hope you fall apart. They hope to see you fall to pieces."

I was astounded. But, I also got one of those large Guy grins across my face, and retorted, "Really. They hope to see me fall apart? Really?"

"Yep, they want you to see your faith fall apart."

"Wow!" I exclaimed in surprise.

To be honest, that was all I needed to hear. My faith was not in jeopardy here. And all I needed to know was that some were watching, so I made it my plan and goal to be even more overt, maybe even obnoxious about how God was on my side more than ever. I make no apologies.

So off I headed, new attitude in place and growing. My new attitude just got a huge dose of fertilizer. You know, sometimes it takes crap to get the seeds off to a great start. In the fields of life, like farming, one must put up with a little dose of fertilizer to grow up healthy and strong. My commitment and faith got a boost that day.

I have never confronted those guys about their hopes to see me crack. I can tell you this, though. I felt absolutely certain that they would never have the chance to watch me do the Humpty Dumpty; I was willing to bet my life on it.

Every once in a while I would hear that some were still watching. With each of those moments I was less astonished than before. Really, I couldn't have cared less. The root that had started was now deeper than ever. The thoughts in my head continued to mature and swirl, altering how I would look at cancer, life, and faith. But, no matter, the rock on which I was setting my foundation for change was an immovable rock.

This Humpty Dumpty wasn't headed for a fall any time soon.

We need to welcome the *supplements* that make our faith and resolve grow, make them our friends. So when you're out there in your own little field called life, take a good look at who may be watching and why. In my field, someone else was watching, someone the others could not see, and he wasn't about to let me down.

FACING YOUR FEARS

Do you think of yourself as a winner? A fighter? We can *talk* all we want about how we would react to this or that, or even cockily say, "I'm not afraid of _____," but frankly I have found these to be empty words until my feet are held to the fire. Then we'll see; then we'll see. I believe that it is only when we stand face to face with our fears that we really earn the right to talk.

Cancer has a way of helping fear rear its ugly head. Is there anyone who is not living with the fear of cancer, diagnosed or not? Today, more than at any other time in our history we are bombarded by stuff related to cancer. New reports on affected percentages of the population keep us up to date on our odds, as if we really want to hear this every night. But there those reports are, often smack dab in the middle of our dinner hour. My wife just loves all the mammogram stuff right at dinner, or maybe some nice footage of someone's colon, followed by the vast array of erectile dysfunction commercials. Isn't that just the frosting on the dinner cake?

Doctors' offices remind us gently and not so gently, "It's time for your testing! You know, at "your age" it's time to have your [pick a body part] scanned, probed, or squeezed to make sure." Thank you very much. Like I need them to tell me I'm over fifty and have yet to have my colon scanned or blown up like a balloon for one of those "new" less invasive examinations. Right. Less invasive. I can see the doctor standing there with a large pin, and me a balloon—BOOM! The next thing I know I'm flying around the room just like a deflating balloon producing all kinds of nasty noises.

How about all of the ads related to the overarching causes of cancer. I think all of the work being done is great. Don't get me wrong. Race for this, walk for that, support this, and participate by all means. But watching it doesn't give us a break either. Like it or not, we're confronted with reminder after reminder, a steady stream from cancer's 24/7 hotline right into our brains.

Can you think of any other disease on the planet that gets as much press? Personally speaking, I have often felt sorry for the many other illnesses that are inflicting huge casualties, with great amounts of human suffering that go unnoticed except by their victims and the families who can do nothing but sit and watch like a bad horror film.

Earlier on I spoke with you about changing my cancer visits into a mission field. What I began to learn was that this was only the first step in a change that was taking hold in my thinking process. When I changed my perspective about the visits, the visits changed. What happened at the visits didn't change; the visits changed.

When I changed the way I viewed the doctors, the doctors didn't change, except if they were faced inwardly with questions about why I was different from the normal patient. For example, while being tested, I focused on the technicians instead of focusing on the test. The list could go on, but you catch my drift. And, on occasion a nurse would ask, or a tech, or a doctor. Why was I still smiling, or happy? Why wasn't I depressed, fearful, or concerned?

Perspective. What do you have the power to change if not your own perspective? A changed perspective gives birth to the potential for powerful "life" change. This is what I was learning. First, as I changed my perspective on my testing or visits, the testing and visits changed in a way that gave me power over them, instead of the visits or testings having power over me.

As this mission field perspective took hold I became more concerned about the people who were supposed to be helping me. I tried to help them, to be friendly. As that change matured I found myself changing the way I looked at myself also. Changing your perspective can bring a health to your health. Little by little, change after change, fears found themselves without a home.

MAYBE HE WON'T KNOW

I found people reacting to this cancer stuff in funny ways. Not that I was laughing at them—don't take it that way—but have you ever gotten the feeling that others thought they knew something you didn't, but you actually did know? How did it make you feel? When it all came out, how did it make them feel when they found out you knew all along? Being a cancer patient is a lot like that. That's what I discovered early on as I attempted to walk through my day as I once had—before I was diagnosed with cancer.

As surprising as it may seem, those of us who have cancer know it. Stating this makes me want to chuckle, as a grin spreads across my face. What I have found most interesting is how others have reacted to my adventure with cancer.

Speaking to those of us who have faced cancer, I recognize that there are many people out there today who genuinely would like to talk to you about it and offer support, but don't know how. In my case, it was not one specific incident that brought this fact home to me. It was in the day-to-day at work. It was in the day-to-day at college, as I attended classes. It was in the day-to-day moments out in the world. If we "look," it is not hard to spot them the people who want to support you but don't know how. They ask leading questions that may be as simple as, "How are you?" but their eyes or body language tell you they want to ask you more. They may start sentences and search for the words that might finish them. It can be as simple as "that" look, or as obvious as the silence created when words cannot be found. They may pass, saying nothing, but you both know that you've just experienced an awkward moment.

You know it's going to be up to us to help them. It's going to be up to us to become more comfortable in our own skin. It should seem pretty clear by now that I am putting it all out there, but just wait, the real gory details are right round the corner. People want to know, and care, and want to let us know they are thinking about us, but they often don't because the topic hits too close to home. Or perhaps an experience prevents them from expressing what they are feeling or would like to say. We are the only people who can help them, pure and simple.

In many cases, I found myself just telling people right out, "Hey, I know I have cancer so it won't come as a surprise to me when you ask about it." It is often up to us to break the ice, open the door, offer them an invitation. We have to let them know that while it may be uncomfortable for us both, we are glad they want to know and ask.

I know it can be very personal. Part of the problem is that we spend so much time walking around covered with neat little facades. I know this demands that we as cancer patients be willing to be honest with ourselves first. Only to the degree that we have faced ourselves in the mirror of this new life will we be freed to expose ourselves to others, helping them, and helping ourselves.

None of us likes to be exposed because it leaves us vulnerable. But what if you turned that thinking on its head? What if you allowed yourself to become comfortable in your exposure? Instead of leaving us vulnerable, I believe it makes us stronger and less vulnerable. I believe strength, real strength, rests in the security of knowing I am comfortable in my exposure, because I am comfortable with who I am. We are only left with thoughts of vulnerability when we are uncomfortable in who we are.

I know that it demands a good hard look in the mirror. But, in the end you will be equipped in unimaginable ways to endure whatever may come next and be provided with the strength necessary so that others will be freed as well. I can't tell you how many people, mostly men, came and spoke to me once we let down our false fronts and got all that other crap out of the way. But it took me looking right at them and telling them, "I already know I have cancer," to dismantle the wall that stood between us.

Openness is paramount. Letting people know you are no more afraid to talk about it than you are of your cancer is critical to opening the door for dialogue. So many of us know someone with cancer today. I always hoped that if they became comfortable talking with me it might just help them talk to others as well. What I found was that soon they would begin to ask all kinds of questions about how I knew, or if I knew. What did it feel like? How was this treatment or that treatment, or what did I think about getting tested? MOST importantly, you will be able to offer them direction when they are wondering about a situation they feel is going on in their own bodies. You can offer hope in the face of fear. You can offer help as they too take their first steps on this journey.

I know we're not doctors, but that doesn't mean we can't still be a damn good road map. Just hang a sign around your neck that says, "I know I have cancer and am not afraid to talk about it." And wait and see what happens.

Chapter 10

To my SHAME

If you had to pick which is worse, scars or wounds, what would you pick?

To my shame some of the deepest wounds I have left behind are NOT carried by me. This seems like as good a time as any—just before heading into my description of the second surgery—to take a break from the story to talk about how Liz and I were dealing with all this junk. We all have "our" ways, don't we?

Liz and I have been married for 26 years, and there is such a thing as male intuition. My intuition has repeatedly told me that this has been much tougher on Liz than it has been on me. Liz wasn't emotional, at least not around me. She didn't suffer with bouts of depression or anxiety—as far as I know. I never saw that in her, and I would have noticed. But, this was much harder on Liz, and still is.

Here are the facts. We've experienced six plus years of ups and downs. But it's when Loyola calls when we least expect it—BAM—that I can instantly see, feel, and hear a change in her demeanor. It doesn't take a rocket scientist to figure out your wife. You know, when you can see the little things, like posture, tone, demeanor, or changed levels of energy or enthusiasm. Plain and simple—that spark is missing from her eye along with the smile from her face. It doesn't take long to miss them when they're gone. I've had six years to hone my skills of detection, and it just happened again with that infamous phone call from Scene One.

We never talked about the cancers much. We made sure that decisions and key appointments were attended by us both, but we never sat and talked about its impact on us or our family. To my shame, I don't recall asking Liz how she was feeling. It's not my style not to ask; I just don't remember doing so. If I didn't, it's not because I didn't care. It's because of my approach to this whole thing. Even people at work would question my cavalier style of moving through these events. I'm sure it's one of my coping mechanisms, but that doesn't mean it was supposed to be a coping mechanism for Liz as well. "So where do we go from here?" was simply a question neither one of us ever asked.

Knowing what I know now, I wished I had taken steps to cross this divide. One of the ways I tried to impart strength and help others was by demonstrating my own inner strength. But that only ensured I wouldn't ask some of the needed questions. I wanted no visible perception of weakness on my part.

Honestly, I'm touching on this subject because it needs to be said. Sometimes we are not the ones that come out of this the worse for wear. Sometimes it is our loved ones or close friends who come through these things worse than we do. As I see it, these types of situations demand that we shift our focus 180 degrees. We've talked about that together already. I admit it can be hard, but it's still true. I wasn't using a 180 degree shift. I was telling myself that if this works for me—being cavalier, joking, etc.—then I'm sure it's working for Liz just fine. Don't even ask me if I talked to our son Dan. The answer would be No! I don't believe I did, to my shame.

This section is short and not so sweet for reasons that should be obvious. I can't write about what I don't know. I am unfamiliar with what my wife went through on the inside. What she thought or how much she worried is beyond my knowledge. I don't know if she even worried about my mortality. I don't know, because to my shame I didn't ask. I know I've said that already, but it needs repeating because I need to hear it again. I don't recall her telling me about what was worrying her. That's not her style. She would put on a strong face because that's part of who she is. I hope she was confiding in someone, but I don't know that either.

So what to make of this? I suggest we allow our loved ones to be open and honest with us—even when we don't want to hear it, and they would just as soon not say it. Truth is, they didn't choose this anymore than we did. So together we need to work to create an environment that will allow our loved ones or friends to be open and honest with us about how this is impacting them. These impacts need to be dealt with. Good or bad, angry or sad—all parties need to be free to express themselves. How they are thinking and feeling is just as valid as what we might be feeling or thinking. Everyone can benefit from this openness; it is emotionally and physically therapeutic.

I believe that harboring these feelings and things bind us up. If our loved ones are allowed to be honest, they may even admit that they hate you for coming down with cancer, even though they know, rationally speaking, it wasn't your choice. They may harbor ill feelings as they too watch their dreams—your dreams together—come crashing down.

A key part of freedom for all involved is open expression. Team work will win the day in the face of vast pressures. But teamwork only happens well if there is communication. Talking about real fears and frustrations can strengthen our ability to help one another. Open communication can let them help you be free to be you. More importantly, it can help them be free to be who they are!

We need to help everyone thrown out of balance by a diagnosis of cancer to find their balance again. It may require some added attention, and that's not always easy to muster. But, take this from someone who knows, sometimes the person with the illness has it easier than the person who does not. We often have permission to just "be," while they are forced to fill all of the voids created by this situation on top of all that they may be feeling already.

So if you were to ask me which is worse, I would tell you that I have the scars, but it is Liz who carries the wounds! In a spirit of revelation I've asked Liz to write her own experiences and thoughts. It seems only fitting that her voice should finally be heard.

Chapter 11

Liz speaks OUT

Cancer. Great!!

I remember the day as if it were yesterday. I am a school secretary.
My job requires that I begin work at the beginning of August and
finish in the middle of June. I was sitting at my desk that mid-
August day when Guy called me in the afternoon to let me know
that he had had his PSA level tested and that it was elevated.
Not being too familiar with terms associated with male cancers, I
wasn't exactly sure what an elevated PSA level meant. Little did I
realize what was to follow.

The year 2004 was NOT a good year for our family. My mom became ill in April and passed away in June. I was still numb and grieving her death when my husband announced this new chapter in our life together. Here I was, trying to figure out how to live without my mother and how her absence was to reshape our lives, and now cancer threatened to take away my husband, too. CANCER—great!

So we started down the path that would reveal both testicular and prostate cancer in my husband. Guy is not the type of person that goes to doctors. He even refused to go to a doctor when I knew that his finger had been broken on the job because it was bent in ways it shouldn't be. He's stubborn and determined. I knew that if he was going to a doctor for an elevated PSA level this must be serious.

Women know all sorts of things about their bodies and the cancers that could someday present themselves. This is because women talk and read and communicate. Men—not so much! When it comes to illnesses of the "male" type, most men bury their heads in the sand, ignore the problem, and hope it will go away.

My husband was no different. I was NOT very happy when I found out that he had ignored the symptoms of testicular cancer for TWO years before telling me or doing anything about it. I couldn't yell at him. We couldn't go back. Done was done. So off we went on this new adventure. What else are you supposed to do?

I believe that women are inherent caregivers. We put others before ourselves. We put away our feelings in order to take charge and take care of those we love. Unfortunately, in this case, I could do NOTHING but be there for the doctor appointments and surgeries and recoveries. I couldn't take away the pain of biopsies or surgeries or follow-up visits. I could only be there physically and provide emotional support.

I remember driving my husband to his class at the Christian university he was attending in the northern suburbs the day after his release from the hospital. I did this ONLY because the university had a stupid rule that said if you missed a class, ONE HALF TO ONE WHOLE GRADE POINT WAS DEDUCTED FROM YOUR FINAL GRADE! No exceptions—NOT EVEN FOR CANCER!! I had never heard of anything so ridiculous in my life—and this was supposed to be a CHRISTIAN university. Unbelievable! To this day, I will not support or encourage anyone or anything associated with this particular institution of higher learning. Someday, someone will have to stand before God Almighty and be held accountable for their "Christian" actions in deciding to penalize their students for things in life that are beyond the students' control. Gee—I'm facing a cancer right now that might take my life, but don't pray for me or support me; just deduct that grade point because I missed ONE class! My husband had never missed a class in three years. It is our hope that policies such as theirs are not the norm.

We were surrounded by loving and caring family members, friends, and co-workers. You know you are loved when you can sit down with family and friends and discuss medical terms, anatomical descriptions, surgery experiences, and then have coffee!!

Guy required two surgeries, six weeks apart. One surgery was around Labor Day and one was the second week of October. The first surgery was a day surgery, and Guy came through with flying colors. It was actually interesting to see him on Vicodin, because he is not one for medications. The second surgery was more intense and scary. It was a very long day and my dad and brother and sister-in-law sat with me in the Loyola University Medical Center surgical waiting room. After the surgery and once Guy was assigned a room, we were allowed to go in and visit him. My sister-in-law, who is a nurse, commented that he really looked wonderful. I wasn't so sure. Long days followed until he was released and we were allowed to come home.

It's interesting—our world was consumed by worry and surgeries and recovery and still the real world kept spinning. Our son Daniel continued to go to school, although I still feel guilty because he was only 16 and I felt that I did not sufficiently parent him through this experience. I hope he realizes that I knew he was (and still is) a great young man and that at this particular time in our lives his dad needed me more.

My co-workers at school did a wonderful job of filling in for me. This is not easy. Our office is extremely busy, so when one of us is absent, it only creates a burden for those remaining. I was gone for four days, which was a record for me. I'm never gone that long. When I returned, my desk was filled with encouraging notes and gift cards for restaurants, so that I would not have to cook. I was deeply touched by the support of my co-workers. They are awesome!

For better or worse, recovering from surgery requires care. I am a caring person. I had no trouble caring for Guy and taking care of those things that needed taking care of. Helping with catheters and tubes and emptying urine bags and keeping things clean was fine, but I was surprised when, due to the way the catheter and tube and bag were situated I had to sleep on the other side of the bed to what I was accustomed—and found I couldn't sleep! Everything felt different and uncomfortable and weird. Isn't that silly? I can only imagine how different and uncomfortable and weird Guy felt.

I am grateful for the God-given strength of my husband. He was the one who had to go through this experience, and he made it easier for me with his humor and confidence. Thankfully, we have come through this experience together. Once you have shared something like this, you are stronger both individually and as a couple. As he always told me, "Life will never be boring!" Little did I know!!

Chapter 12

Suddenly you find yourself, your family, your home, and all you have known lying directly in the path of a vast army.

There they stand marshaled into attack formations, weapons at the ready, each face telling a story—a story of capture and cruelty, a story of victory. Carried by a strong south wind, the dust from their chariots and horsemen fills your nostrils. Dead ahead is a new destiny. One not of your choosing, one impossible to escape.

You will resist as best you can, but soon you too will fall. Maybe it is best to fall? Your mind swirls through a range of emotions, heart pounding. You scramble to ensure your family will be safe, but in the distance the unavoidable marches ever closer. Your eyes flash quickly back and forth between the present and your future. Soon the ground begins to shake at their advance. Soon, and it will be soon, the mighty King Nebuchadnezzar will add your people to his massive slave population. Soon, with nothing but the bare clothes on your back, you will be carried off against your will into captivity.

Conquests like this were common in ancient times. Enslavement was common. What I find most interesting are the tactics employed once the slaves reached "their new home."

The problem with slaves is their will. Docile slaves don't cause problems and are easily controlled. So what's my point with all of this? The point is this: if you want to control a person's will to fight back you need to erase their memories of home. The Babylonians were experts in this.

When captives reached Babylon they were separated from what was familiar—their homes and hometowns, their very history on their land. As strangers in Babylon they were also given Babylonian names to erase the connection with their former identity. But it didn't stop there. They were forced to wear Babylonian clothing and eat only Babylonian food and drink. Only the customs of the Babylonians were to be practiced.

Imagine yourself as one of those living in captivity in Babylon. Systematically, effectively, and with precision—stolen was WHO you once were. Stolen was WHAT you once knew. Stolen was HOW you once lived. Stolen was WHERE you once lived. YOU had been erased! YOU WERE GONE!

Quite interesting the way captivity works, wouldn't you say?

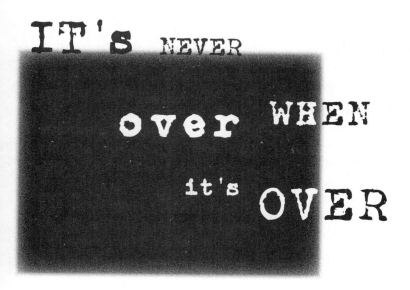

Chapter 13

IT'S NEVER over WHEN it's OVER

Liz and I hopped in the car and headed off to Loyola Medical Center.

The sun isn't up yet; we were to arrive bright and early. It's been six weeks. We walked in the entrance and began the sign-in paperwork. No day surgery this time. I was heading for a three-day stay. The wonders of drugs don't permit me to explain some parts of what's coming because the drugs erase them from your memory. So I'll give it to you as I remember it.

A nice woman seated in a chair in an oddly shaped cubical admissions area did our paperwork. From there we proceeded to a changing area, but honestly, that part is rather foggy. I know I was asked to put on a gown but don't remember doing it. I remember lying in a bed in the surgical waiting area after changing. Liz was still with me at this point. She was reading a magazine she had brought with her.

While in surgical waiting, various nurses, techs, and the anesthesiologist paid me a visit. It's not like I was popular; I was just one more patient on a long list of patients. Even so, they treated me great. The nurses took my vitals. The techs drew some blood, I think, along with doing an EKG (electrocardiogram). They wanted to make sure my heart was OK. Funny. I had run marathons, trained with weekly run totals of 45–50 miles and maintained heart rates of 170 beats per minute for over an hour and a half. My heart was strong. Just give it a listen. They assured me everything was normal. What a surprise! Duh.

Then I was visited by the anesthesiologist, and it was funny to me. I had to stick out my tongue and let them look down my throat. They wanted to make sure they could get their tube down there. He didn't take much time; it was more like an introduction, "Hi, I'm doctor so-and-so." Everything checked out OK. Liz sat bedside and we cracked some jokes. What the heck, why not? Just because you're having surgery doesn't mean you have to be a dud.

Can't say for sure how long we waited there. Then I was moved again. This time Liz could not go with. She was informed that the surgery would take about three hours, if all went according to plan. They directed her to the surgical waiting room. I told her I'd see her in a little bit. Sadly, I don't remember if we kissed. We're not much on public displays. I'm not much on blowing things out of proportion. Everything was going to be fine. What's the big deal?

Soon I found myself in another waiting area, but I don't remember being moved. Here's where the IV was put in. They would use it to administer the drugs for knocking me out, and in the event something went wrong. For those of you who have had an IV, great. For those of you who haven't, here's how it goes.

First, they place a tourniquet around your upper arm. Then they ask you to make a fist and squeeze. This causes the veins in your arm to swell with blood, making them stand out. By the way, nurses and doctors alike have all loved my veins. I am easy to stick. Once they find the spot they like right near the inside of your elbow area, they warn you that it will pinch a little. Then with a push a hollow needle is inserted into your vein just under the skin. Once they're sure they have a good location with good flow they tape the IV needle down to your arm. The needle has a plastic gizmo attached to it—I know, a very medical term. With that in place they can infuse your body with various things throughout the surgery, during recovery, or during your stay. It does sting, but great nurses and techs make it almost painless with no extra bleeding around the site, which would result in black and blue discoloration like a bruise.

Once the IV was in place, I was soon visited by a young man with brown hair. I know he had his name on his jacket, but I don't remember who he was, if I knew at all. All I remember was him standing at the foot of the bed, clipboard in hand, stethoscope professionally hanging around his neck; that's it. I don't remember what we talked about. I don't remember them administering anything into my IV to knock me out. No warning. No fuzzies like the last time. I don't even remember everything going dark. I was listening to a young man standing at the foot of my bed, white coat and all—and then I was not.

The next thing I knew I was in a hospital room. Not post-recovery but a regular patient room. It was about five-thirty in the evening. Hours, not sure how many, were gone. There sat Liz. She was seated to my left in the hospital room, watching over me like a sentinel, protecting what she held dear. I am truly a lucky man. At this point, I don't remember if I was in a recovery room or not. But there I was, my new home away from home.

For those of you who are less squeamish, here's what they did to me in surgery, the part I don't remember, of course. This is only a rough sketch, real rough. And remember, I'm not a doctor. I can't tell you precisely what happened. I have often wanted to go back to the hospital and watch the procedure done. I haven't asked or gotten the chance yet. Maybe I'll ask at my next visit; it's coming up soon.

So here's what I know. The order of my details may be a little off, but you'll get the picture. Part of the procedure involves putting a catheter into your bladder. The prostate gland is located just below your bladder, and your urinary canal runs smack dab through the middle of it leading out of your body through, well, you know. An incision is made just below your belly button running to the top of your pubic bone, about three inches in total. Now, let me just say at this time that there are tons of nerves that run through all of the stuff that control a man's ability to have erections and such. It is important that the doctor remove the gland while at the same time doing as little damage to those nerves as possible. That's why they warn you that a byproduct of prostate surgery can be permanent impotence! That's why most men shy away from getting checked in the first place. Dumb move men, dumb move.

So, that said, the surgeon cuts through your skin first and your abdominal muscles next. That allows the surgeon to enter your abdomen and expose the gland. He (or she) removes the prostate gland protecting as many nerves as possible during the surgery, and then inserts a Foley catheter. Time will tell how well the surgeon did and what the outcome may be. We'll talk about that later.

So, there I was in my room lying in bed with a small j-tube coming out of my lower abdominal area. This tube works like a drain to remove additional bleeding from the internal surgical site. I also had a three inch incision running from just below my belly button to just above my, well, you know. The incision was stapled closed. Accompanying these goodies was a catheter to drain my bladder and protect the plumbing changes from surgery and an IV line. That's that. Surgery number two complete.

When I first awoke I really had to urinate. But, because I'm an adult, and there stood the nurse, and there sat Liz, I wasn't willing. So I tightened my bladder muscles and squeezed. That took care of that. Picture a long car ride with no rest stop in sight. I could pinch off the catheter hard enough to not go. But that was only going to last just so long. I remember the nurse saying, "You need to just relax and let yourself go." It took the nurse to give me permission! That was weird, and I remember it being weird. Plus my wife and my nurse were both there. My wife in the chair, the nurse holding the plastic container connected to the catheter to check for output. Tell me that's not weird and that it's not going anywhere night or day for two weeks. That's fourteen days—three hundred thirty six hours. Well, you get it.

Question. Have you ever had a friend who just kept hanging around when you're hoping inside they would just go somewhere, anywhere? Of course the catheter and bag didn't leave; it just kept hanging around. Hanging is a good word. It's OK to laugh. Actually, it is kind of funny, but I didn't think so then.

That same evening, not long after getting to my room, I was visited by my brother and sister-in-law, and my father-in-law. They were greeted by my smiling face. I only mention it, because I can still hear my sister-in-law, a life-long registered nurse say, "Wow, does he look good! He's not supposed to look this good coming out of surgery." Ah, the wonder of connections. I also have kept myself fit. Your fitness level makes a huge difference when you go through surgery, or are recovering from surgery.

Soon their visit would end. Soon Liz headed home. I'm sure she was exhausted, but she never showed it, or told me. I don't recall asking. Ask her and she'll tell you, "I was just doing what I was supposed to do." She reminds me often, "My job is to take care of you and Dan." And she truly does.

With no place to go, I lay there and watched as the evening faded into night. Nights at hospitals are not restful, but I slept off and on. Pain drugs can truly be wonderful. Normally after this type of surgery they give you morphine. I've heard stories of men having a gizmo that would let them push a button when they felt they needed pain relief. I didn't get a gizmo, but I didn't need it either. I was only on morphine briefly and have no recollection of it or its effects. From there you graduate down to pain meds that don't carry with them the addictive properties of morphine.

Here's a revelation: when it comes to stuff like this, I don't give myself many options. The goal is simple: return to life as I knew it ASAP, no matter what. I tend to be tough on myself at times. But as my pops always said, "The body is made for work." There's no going easy. I tend to think I'm the one giving the orders here.

It didn't take long for the night nurses to arrive. Shift change is a hectic time. I've found the typical shift is twelve hours, and shift change usually occurred between six or seven, AM or PM, pick one. What's interesting is how some of the night nurses in particular would come in your room and needed little or no lighting to do their work. That was really cool. It sure beat the alternative, when the nurse would come in and turned on what seemed to be every light possible. Visits happened like clockwork. There was little sleeping. Mostly it was being checked by this person and that and then trying to fall asleep again, only to be awakened again a few hours later. While it may sound like I didn't appreciate all the interruptions, it was OK. You don't want to bite the hand that feeds you, if you know what I mean. The first night was the worst. Trying to get used to the catheter wasn't fun at all. Resting was not a word I would necessarily use to describe how I slept, or what it felt like to just lie there. They did great pain management; I had no pain.

Another thing the night brought with it was the compression gizmos they put on your legs. They ran from your foot to your knee. They were hooked up to an air supply which, in turn, would inflate and deflate these bag-like things to push the blood in and out of your legs. They are used to prevent the possibility of blood clots. Added to everything else, they made sleeping interesting.

The first day brought little challenges. The greatest challenge was having a roommate. Mine talked too loud, didn't use the curtain at times when it would have been welcomed, and watched cooking shows—all day long. It can be boring, so bring a book! He never turned the TV off, day or night. I suppose I could have said something, but I tried focusing on other things. Besides, that's not my style. We didn't talk. It wasn't one of those, "Oh gee, what are you in for..." moments. I really wasn't interested.

Each day's events included visits by a rotation of interns. Loyola is a teaching hospital. You guessed it. Everybody and their brother or sister might come through the door at one time or another. The interns were the most interesting. "Hello Mr. Beck, how are you feeling today?"

"Fine."

"Oh, would you mind if WE ALL had a look?"

Sounds like a question, but we all know it's not. Back go the blankets. Gee it's kind of like show and tell, except you're the show! Tubes coming out of various places already described, a magnificent incision, staples and all my glory—so to speak—right out there for the entire world to see. The only blessing is that by now it had happened so often that I didn't care anymore, like I could go anywhere anyway. Captivity, yeah, captivity, that rings a bell, I'd seen this done before. Captivity. In time, short walks in the hall would bring diversion to the constant prison of my bed and the TV that was always annoyingly on.

Day one also brought with it a funny plastic clown machine. Following surgery, they also worry about pneumonia setting in. So the solution for that is to blow in the plastic tube connected to this clown thing. You're supposed to blow hard enough to make the ball inside pop up on scale of measurements. They wanted to measure lung capacity and force me to use my lungs in a way that prevents pneumonia. The clown on the machine is more for the kids. All I could keep thinking is, I run marathons, and you think my lungs need a work out? They gave their orders; so many repetitions per set and so many sets each day. I did as I was told and saw it as just one more challenge. Maybe, just maybe, I could blow that ball right out of the top of the clown's head. Those machines are really stupid looking with a clown on them.

The two remaining days were not unlike what has already been described, except for drug dosages that decreased. Oh, I made that pain medication mistake just once. I felt really good, so I told the nurse it wouldn't be necessary to continue the pain med I was on. It wasn't long before I found out I needed more pain management care than I thought. When she came back I apologized for thinking I knew better, and she did her thing. Soon I felt great once more. Well, how else was a guy supposed to learn?

Nearing the end of my stay meant that the j-tube would come out. Once they feel that the surgical site has sufficiently healed and drained you don't need the tube. Listen, when they say, "You're only going to feel *a little* discomfort." Tell 'em "yeah, right!" It wasn't the last time I would hear those words.

I'm not exactly sure how that tube is fastened at the site inside of you, but pulling out this four or five inch long very thin tube was uncomfortable. Sometimes I feel like we should get something in trade; like tit for tat, seems childish as I say it. I know that the person performing the procedure was just doing their job, and meant me no ill will, but this stuff sure seems awfully one-sided at times. There was a sharp sting when he first pulled, followed by this weird pulling, sliding sensation. Then it was out.

But something happened during my stay that was far more interesting than all the junk I have been describing. As it would happen, one evening one of the hospital's chaplains paid me a visit. Man, I knew the drill forwards and backwards. There I lay, Liz seated in the chair next to the bed. A knock on the door and in she walks, white chaplain coat and all. Per the drill she begins by saying "Hello" to the patient and then to any family or friends who may be present. This is followed by a shake of the hand when appropriate and soon by asking whether the patient needs anything, or if the chaplain can be of any help.

But this was different; I was the Guy in the bed. Interesting. There I was, and all I kept thinking was, "How can I get her out of here?" I knew how she felt cold-calling and all. I was doing a chaplaincy internship rotation when all this got started. I knew how little people seemed to welcome you or even care that you stopped by. But I also knew how it felt when they welcomed your visit! Initially, I wanted to send her off with a "Thanks for coming, I'm fine." But Liz must have known. She gave me one of those looks. A glare really, and I welcomed the chaplain to sit. We shared. I talked with her about my experiences with chaplaincy. I asked about hers. We prayed together. It was a blessing. What a kick in the head.

Because of her visit, just as that older man at Copley was there for me during my internship, I understood better what it meant to show someone appreciation. She could have skipped my room or sensed that I wasn't interested. She didn't have to come in, but she CHOSE to come in. She wanted to give care, and find out if I was OK. I learned that evening from a hospital bed that I, too, needed care.

This visit would shape the way in which I would look for ways to receive care, and also to offer care to those who came to visit me. Doctors, nurses, and staff of every variety became a new opportunity for expressions of gratitude, grateful for all they were doing for me, as well as being an opportunity to ask them, "How are you doing today?" Sometimes we are so quick to say, "Well, it's their job, isn't it?" or, "They're getting paid, aren't they?"

Finally, my release day arrived. Three days down the tubes. Ha-ha. I was going home. Everything had gone better than planned. I was on the mend. From the moment the nurse told us I was being discharged it felt like an eternity. Eventually, at about 5:30 PM I was wheeled out to the car, "have catheter and bag, will travel." Gingerly, I got into the car and sat down. The evening sky was bright, but now I was going to have to figure out how all this was going to work out at home.

A CATHETER IS AN INTERESTING BEAST

Adorned in my new baggy pants we headed back home. Like a .357 revolver I strapped that catheter bag to my leg. Unfortunately they don't give you holsters for these things. But, open carry was just out of the question. Call it vanity or pride, I didn't want everyone to know.

What I haven't told you up till now was how I ended up at college in the first place. As a young man I dreamt of one day going to seminary for a divinity degree, but in order to do that I needed a bachelor's degree as part of seminary entrance qualifications. So I headed out to Ann Arbor, Michigan to begin that process. That experience only lasted three days; I was simply not prepared for college at that time. But, the desire never left my spirit. Twenty years and many jobs later the desire to attend seminary was rekindled by some friends who suggested I give it another go. This time, instead of heading off to a different state to get a bachelor's degree, it was suggested I attend a local university in the northern suburbs. They had just the type of program that would work well for me as a working adult. This brings us to where we are today. I was in my last year of studies at this time.

All this makes me ask the "what-if" questions. What if the thought of seminary had never come to mind? What if I had let that first disappointing experience rule my thinking? What if my friends had never encouraged me to chase a dream? Twenty years in between is a long time. And then you consider: if each of these events had altered my dream of seminary I would never have ended up here, back at college, doing an internship, finding out I had cancers. There were connections all along, as I see it.

Anyway, as Liz has already told you, this university had a strict policy on attendance. I would attend class once or twice a week depending on how many classes I was taking. The courses ran year round. Each twelve-week course was packed into five weeks. Typically you were able to finish a four-year program in three, which is nice when you're an older working student trying to get done. I was enrolled in two courses at this time.

I enjoyed my studies and considered myself a dedicated student. I had informed the professor about my impending surgery and turned in early any papers that were due. I also asked a class friend, Jeremy, to tape-record the lecture. The professor was a wonderful woman who knew of the policy for absences. The standard had been set. According to school policy, miss one class, or even a half of one class, and a deduction of one half grade to one full grade was to be deducted from your final grade. I had never missed a class in three years until that night, the night before my surgery. I had never arrived so much as minutes late. The professor and I talked about my impending absence, and she appreciated the difficulties of my situation.

She also expressed concerns for my wellbeing, which was nice. But, her hands were tied. My final grade was an A- . The half grade deduction due to my absence was applied. This was the best I could do based on policy. From our discussions her frustration with the policy was evident, but policy is policy, right? I wish to thank her for her understanding, if she were to ever read this.

After missing the mid-week class I often thought about my upcoming second course on Saturday from my hospital bed. There was no way I was going to let them dock me again if humanly possible. I was discharged about 5:30 PM on Friday, and on Saturday morning at 9 AM I was in class, catheter, bag, and all. Liz drove; I wasn't cleared for driving. What a blast.

That class was led by an awesome human being and professor. I wish to thank him as well. He knew of the policy and he knew of my surgery. He was shocked that I had even shown up, but he knew why. In time I was whipped and really glad to be heading back home. I was the recipient of his kindness on that day.

When I told a pastor friend of mine about the policy he called the university. All they could assure him of was that they were terribly sorry, but policy is policy. You know. Our hands are tied. He was furious at their insensitivity. I never missed another class, thank you very much.

Let me just say, before lightening this up a lot. Policy is policy. Grace is grace. Sometimes amidst life there are places where we are trapped by the policies we create, rather than being led by the grace that we know is best. Maybe my friend's call or a word from the professors may have helped to change this policy, but I can't say for sure because I don't know if they ever changed it. But I can hope. All I can say is, they taught me more than they may ever know.

After that trip to class I didn't go anywhere for a few days, and that was a good thing. Just moving around the house was tricky enough with the catheter, let alone the incision. So there I sat, mastering the craft of emptying the bag. Each time, I would have to wash the bag. My wife got to help with some of that. The hours click by. At night, my wife reminded me. Because of the bag we had to change the side of the bed we each slept on. My wife couldn't sleep. It was the wrong side of the bed. Give it a try sometime.

As the days marched on I learned better how to set things up for sleeping. Where to put the bag, how to position the tubing, to turn or not to turn, watching out for that darn tube. Last thing you wanted was to kink it. So, you do more dozing than sleeping because your mind is always conscious of its presence.

During the day it was somewhat easier, but it was always there. Sometimes it would slip from how I had it fastened to my mid-thigh. As it fell the tube would slide out, running into the inflated bulb on the end in your bladder giving it a little tug. I'd react as quickly as I could, grabbing the bag and sliding some of the tube back in to take the tension off. That's how each day went.

Beyond going to my mid-week class I did nothing but homework and watch TV. I drove myself to the mid-week class. Only Jeremy and the professor knew what had gone on. I sat in class like I didn't have a catheter bag lashed to my leg. During the break I went into one of the stalls in the men's room and emptied the bag, returning to class like it was just a normal trip to the bathroom.

After about the first week I added in some short walks, bag and all, to my daily routine. It was just nice to get outside. I thought about whether this was overdoing it, but walking helped me think I was back on track.

At about the week and a half mark I had a visit with Dr. Frank. I was having some pus-like discharge around the catheter so I called the doctor. He advised me to keep the area clean, and that I should rest easy. I just wanted that thing out. It hurt. It was itchy. It was TIME! So I did the macho thing; I begged him to see me and take it out. "Two weeks." That was his response. It needed to be in for two full weeks so all involved could fully heal. In my head I knew that would be the response. It made perfect sense, but . . .

WATCHFUL WAITING

That's what they called it. The typical follow-up after my orchiectomy (testicle removal) was radiation treatments. I learned this as part of a follow-up visit after the surgery. One more doctor. Another urologist or cancer specialist, not sure which, a woman doctor this time, along with the usual physical exam. More decisions.

She was the first doctor to lay out for me what the follow-up procedures would be. She spelled it out: a general dose of radiation treatments pointed at my lower abdomen. I remember thinking she told me once per day for a month, but now I'm not sure, so let's just go with radiation treatments, plural. I was assured that this was considered a normal course of follow-up treatment. The goal was simple, kill with radiation what may have been missed by the knife. Sounds like a plan.

The thing is, when you get a general dose of radiation shot at your lower abdomen like this it can affect a lot of other things in that general area, like your bladder or rectum. Plus, they told me that I would have a ten percent chance of one day getting leukemia or lymphoma as a byproduct of the radiation treatments. I wasn't a fan, so I asked the doctor if there were other options. She advised that another follow-up treatment would be a series of CT scans over YEARS, but you must be diligent about keeping up on them. She really stressed that.

Having completed the prostate surgery, it was also time for a follow-up visit back at Loyola. Dr. Frank met with me per the usual routine. Then it came time to talk about follow-up treatments. The follow-up to prostate surgery was radiation treatments. There I was, like a bad flashback, confronted with decisions about radiation again. Dr. Frank assured me that radiation was the norm, and that would be that. It's kind of like added insurance, nothing to worry about. But then I brought up the whole leukemia and lymphoma stuff I had been told. That was uncomfortable but needed asking. He assured me once more that I didn't have anything to worry about. But I asked, "So if I don't want to be radiated, what other choices do I have?"

"Well, you could undergo a series of CT scans over years. We call it, 'watchful waiting.'" There it was.

The usual procedure for the scans went like this: the first year would be scans every three months; year two would be scans every four months; year three, every six months. Then you have scan once a year with a chest x-ray in between for two more years. Again, I might have some details a little fuzzy. If you want an exact procedure description, ask an expert. Don't rely on my memory. I don't recall being told how long this would go on. I thought maybe five years. You hear that five years being cancer free is the number you want to shoot for, then you're good to go.

While the CT scan option wasn't all that enticing from an occurrence standpoint, it still seemed better than the alternative. Either way, I am still living with the chance of a reoccurrence. But, risking leukemia or lymphoma, not good! No thanks! I wasn't willing to take that chance on radiation treatments, so I declined radiation.

Here's the thing. When I asked the doctor what they would do should the cancers associated with the testicular surgery show up, they told me they would give me radiation treatments anyway. "So, let me get this straight. If I don't get treatments now I won't run the risk of getting lymphoma or leukemia, and my bladder and rectum, among other things, won't be damaged by the radiation treatments."

"That's correct, but you do realize that if it shows up again it could be much worse." Even so, it seemed like a no brainer to me. I opted for the CT scans. If you are faced with this choice, you'll have to weigh the alternatives in consultation with your doctors. I did what seemed best to me.

This was the first time I would hear the words, "watchful waiting." I told them I didn't have much use for that term. Dr. Frank also reminded me that it was not common to skip the radiation treatments, but as long as I stayed faithful to the scans he was willing to move forward this way.

Oh, there was one more thing: the margins on my tested samples. Part of what they check under the microscope is for a distinct separation between what are healthy cells and abnormal cancer cells. They check the borders of the affected areas for signs of normal cells. They want to remove enough of the affected area so that the entire cancerous area is surrounded by healthy tissue. It's like the old saying, "You've got to take the good with the bad." In my case the cancer of the testicle was "fully encapsulated," as they put it. It was confined entirely within the testicle itself. None of the adjoining connective tissues showed any sign of anything other than normal cells.

The prostate cancer cells seemed to be fully confined to my prostate as well. But, here's what confined means: the thickness of a single sheet of ordinary paper. It would be like drawing an abnormal cell on one side of the paper, and a normal cell on the other, with only the thickness of a piece of paper separating them.

So, did they get it all? That's the $64,000 question. The doc felt confident. His vote didn't really count, but was helpful. My vote was the only one that mattered on that day; mine and Liz's of course. If I believed—believed—he did get it all, then watching and waiting made perfect sense. No radiation.

If I didn't believe, then radiation was the order of the day. But, like I have already told you, "I got connections." That's what I kept believing. It was then that Dr. Frank asked me, "Do you feel confident that we got it all?"

"Yes. I have absolute confidence in the faith that it's all gone." So he wrote his orders and headed out of the room. I was now living in the land of "watchful waiting." The orders included my first CT in the three month rotation, and a blood panel workup.

Hey guys, on your next anniversary see how your wife would like his and her CT scans. I really know how to celebrate an anniversary, now don't I? Anyway, each scan was also accompanied by a panel of blood tests to watch for signs that it had come back. One blood test checks for an elevation of a specific enzyme. It's like giving a man a pregnancy test. An elevation in this enzyme in a man's body is used as a tumor marker.

They're still watching, and I'm still getting CT scans. I still hate the term "watchful waiting." They are still watching, but I'm not waiting. I'm living. It doesn't mean I'm not glad someone is watching. I dutifully follow doctor's orders, one CT and blood panel after another. It's been more than six years now; I've lost count of the CT scans and blood work. Actually, it's not so much losing count as much as never trying to remember in the first place. I can't say I've never wondered though, now so many scans later. Even with the best of intentions, scans like these subject our bodies to many more times the radiation than is probably good. All in the name of prevention. As I write this, I'll be due again shortly. The next appointment is just before the Christmas holidays.

I'm telling you, as I told them, "We need to come up with a different term than "watchful waiting."

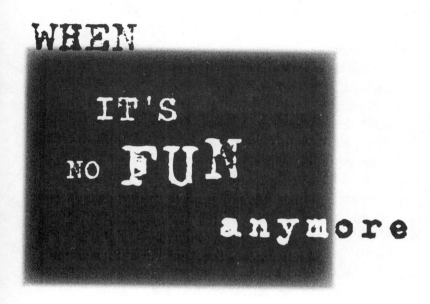

Chapter 14

WHEN IT'S NO FUN anymore

Who hasn't been in that doctor's office?

You know, the office you don't really want to be in, because it's not going to be one of those routine visits where life is good and everything's going to be OK. Who doesn't know what that feels like? You're cool on the outside, but inside you're just waiting for your turn like an inmate sitting on death row. Everyone there knows it's only a matter of time before they call your name.

So I walk in, casually perusing the chairs of Clinic A before I pick mine. We do it instinctively; we do it with calculation.

Mine and Liz's, that is, because she came with me today. Crushed red velvet chairs. Our faces join the faces of the many seated nearby. Sometimes I share a passing glance, but most times I don't. I didn't. Cardinal Bernardin Cancer Center, Clinic A, would become my next home away from home. I knew what brought us there. We all knew what brought us there.

Finally, a nurse calls my name, "Mr. Beck." I pause. "Mr. Beck." Now it's my turn. I get up trying to let everyone know it's no big deal. I'm cool—an easy response. I lift my hand and offer a nice hello. Honestly, I don't think anyone notices. I know we're all sitting there, and we tend to keep track of who seems to be ahead of us, but it's not a good judge, because people are seeing other doctors. But I do it anyway. Inside, the only person I cared about today was me. So, in between my arrival and my turn I paid little attention to anything. I've got this all under control, and I wasn't scared. I was just there because I had to be, needed to be. It was finally "that" time. Even in this, God didn't turn away his head.

I knew my way down that hall, and Liz followed right behind. It's a hall I've walked many times before, but this day was different. In some ways what was about to happen brought unspeakable things to mind. In a sick kind of a way I had been longing for this day. The nurse who preceded us down the hall pointed out the room. By now it felt like I'd been in most of the rooms in that hall. I've lost track of the number of times I've been in them.

But, you can still make a game out of it. Maybe I'll get to go in this room or that one. I haven't been in either of those yet. At least I don't think so. I admit that maybe this is sick, but who hasn't tried to make a game of the morbid as a way to move through times and places in our lives that we'd just as soon forget. Remember, even Jesus prayed for that. ("God, if it be your will, take this cup from me.") Jesus was staring one of those places square in the face and didn't like it any better than us. These times give us a human chance of being just like

Jesus, wanting anything to happen just as long as it wasn't the handwriting on the wall.

So you enter the room, taking that old familiar seat right next to the little nurse's table. No big deal. As usual, they begin by taking your blood pressure and weight, and then ask that same old series of question. How do you feel? Anything bothering you? I sit there exchanging pleasantries with the nurse. That's what I do just to ease the coming tension.

Just that walk down the hall—you can feel your blood pressure going up. Over time I would try to guess what these numbers were going to be compared to the last time. Another game. While we talk, I try to settle myself. You know, take a few calming breaths like most of us do, similar to when we're asked to speak in front of a crowd. I knew one thing for sure, those blood pressure numbers were going to be HIGH. They were. You can tell when they pump on that ball and then listen only to have to pump some more to get it high enough to catch that top number as they let the air out.

As I think about it, even this makes me angry. What gave this place or this disease any right to send my blood pressure sky high? I don't have high blood pressure. I resent the fact that it had this power over me. I would even try to explain the numbers away, as if the nurse might write down a lower, better set of numbers. What a joke.

Today was the day I was getting my catheter removed. Boy, I couldn't wait for that. It had been two weeks, finally. Today was the big day. Once more the nurse enters the room and mentions that it's time. Of course, it's a female nurse. Most of them are. Who cares! Multitudes have already shared in your glory, numbering like the stars in the sky. For those of you who have been down a similar road you know what I mean. Still, in spite of embarrassment, you just want it over and you don't care who does it.

Her advice, or instruction, was simple, "You're going to take a few deep breaths and then push." What the heck—I'm not having a baby here am I?

"Oh, and one more thing . . . you're going to feel a little discomfort when I deflate the little bulb on the end that holds it in your bladder. Oh, and as I pull you need to exhale."

Once again I bolstered my macho resolve and cracked a joke. I wish I could remember exactly what I said, but for you guys out there just think of some slightly off color joke about long rubber hoses; you get the picture. The nurse just gave me one of those looks. Kind of like the one parents give their children when they are less than pleased with them. I told her, "Knowing what you're going to do to me in the next few minutes; well, you gotta laugh," and that was funny. She might as well have just growled her disgust out loud. But I didn't care, because she wasn't me. She was on the easy end of the hose.

"Here we go." I groaned some as she deflated the bulb on the end in my bladder. I should have known better. Boy, when she started pulling it just sickened my stomach, and that foot or so of tubing felt like it was 100 miles long. I wanted to yell, "Deep breaths! A little discomfort! Exhale!" I felt like I was going to throw up. That's how it really felt. I wanted it over and even a millisecond longer than necessary was not going to be soon enough.

Wow, I was really glad when that was over. For those of you who may not know, when you've gone two weeks with a catheter, when it comes out you have to learn how to control your bladder all over again. Zow-wie! It's like potty training for adults. Next thing I knew she whipped out this diaper that looked like it would fit King Kong. As I have said, I'm not a big guy—5'6", 135 lbs. I could have wrapped that thing around me three times. I told her, "No way! What am I supposed to do with that thing? It's not a diaper, it's a table cloth." She still didn't appreciate my humor. Liz just looked at me and rolled her eyes at the nurse. We still get a chuckle out of that visit.

You know, I'm not as dumb as I look. My wife and I had gone to the store before we left for the clinic. I knew diapers were in my future. I stood there and picked out my own diapers. Diapers. Forty-seven years old and diapers—what's wrong with that picture?

The visited ended when the nurse handed me a sheet of paper with what looked like stretching exercises on it. Nice little diagrams of people doing this pose and that.

FOLLOW THE YELLOW BRICK ROAD

So, off I trotted, freed from the catheter and bound by *my* diaper. I was glad to be me again, but the two-year-old version of me again. The nice little poses were Kegel exercises. They're what you're supposed to do to retrain your bladder muscles so you don't keep peeing in your pants.

These exercises were going to be just the ticket! Having been in gymnastics and training as a runner, the thought of doing exercises was not foreign to me; I welcomed them. If this is what it would take, then so be it. So I sat and stood on the floor of our living room and did the exercises over and over again. Our son was in school. Liz was at work. It was just me, and I had lots of time during the day to fill. So I did them, over and over again. And still my bladder muscles would lose their flex, and I would feel that not so nice warm feeling again.

From a bodily perspective I did find the whole thing very interesting. As a kid, you had no real grasp of what you were learning to do, but I knew now. Now I could feel that specific muscle group when it was flexed and holding back my urine. But, I could also feel when there would be a break in my focus and the muscle would relax and urine would be released. I had no idea how much we unconsciously keep our focus on holding that muscle tight.

Just doing the simplest of things like sitting in the sofa demanded I keep alert to tension on that muscle. Walking required more focus. And they told me lifting weighted objects would demand even more. I was pretty much told: Do anything and expect to pee. Doesn't that sound like fun?

One day, two days, on so on, I sat on the floor at home—BY MY SELF—doing these exercises just like they told me. Three days stretched into four. By the fourth day I didn't even like watching myself do these exercises. They didn't seem to be working, or they didn't seem to be aggressive enough. Either way, I felt like a fool doing these things. Yes, some of the things we are expected to do embarrass us. Sometimes, we don't fully understand the benefits of things we are asked to do. They can be downright embarrassing. I needed a different solution. I hated those exercises. They actually made me feel humiliated, rather than just embarrassed. The more I felt forced to do them the more I hated them. Even in secret I hated them.

By now, one of the things I really missed was my runs and just being outside. I'm an outdoors kind of person. So, with the doctor's permission I began going for short walks. Short. Maybe half of a block short. I'm used to running miles, not walking blocks. Quick quiz: when you add exertion to an already weakened bladder what do you think is going to happen? Even so, walking seemed like a good alternative. I would have to concentrate while walking which also provided mild exertion. Walking would demand that I flex my bladder muscle and hold it flexed under mild exertion. Sounded like a plan. But, me being me—a phrase I like to use when I choose to deviate from what I'm told to do—I turned the walks into exercises for my bladder and threw out those sheets of paper on which the bladder exercises had been copied.

To walk simple short distances like a half a block or so was no problem, but if you want to really strengthen your muscles, any of them, you need to put them under greater pressure over longer periods of time. So I would calculate how well I thought I was doing. I kept track of duration, how long it would take to walk a given distance without peeing, and control, my sense of the ability to keep the focused attention necessary to not pee in my pants. Then I would walk farther than I knew I should.

Until you have to focus on your bladder control, you just don't have a clue as to what it takes. As I walked, I had to keep one part of my brain engaged to keep the muscle tight. During the walks it was easy at first. So I met success with lengthening the walks. I needed to walk past my comfort zone. Some days it was all good; other days, well, not so good. It was really interesting to feel and figure out how trained your mind needs to be on this. As you can guess, when you choose to walk farther than you should, sooner or later the inevitable happens.

Day by day I went farther. I was becoming me again. In case you were wondering—I DID NOT WEAR A DIAPER FOR THESE WALKS! That forced me to really buckle down and concentrate. That was the only way I could insure I would really dig in my heels. I faced it head on. And I was not about to lose.

Maybe this wasn't a good idea. Don't tell your doctor I told you to tackle it this way. I'm not recommending you use my method, but it worked for me. And if you do, I would recommend that you pay attention to clothing colors. When you get some colors wet, it really becomes noticeable. Some colors are better if you happen to pee while walking in public.

Once the walks were under control I added some weight lifting. Walks strengthened my long-term control. Weights would sharpen up my short-term control with heavier objects. This dual approach was just the ticket for me. This has served me well for many years now. But, on occasion, when I am really tired or tired and sick, weaker in some way, I can still feel that momentary lapse in my concentration. Guess what happens then?

DILATE THIS!

You know, it's funny how some things "go." On the surface everything seemed to be OK, but over time, weeks maybe, I began to notice that when I urinated, the stream was more constricted and it took more effort to empty my bladder. It was concerning, yes, but when you have just come through the kind of surgery I had you often don't know what is normal or not. Most times doctors offer you a list of typical things to watch for, but we really don't expect them to name every last thing to watch for, do we?

I was grateful that the catheter was a thing of the past, grateful that my walks were getting longer and turning into short jogs, grateful that my bladder control was returning to normal; all systems seemed to be on the mend. Except, except that nagging part of my brain that kept reminding me that my flow felt really bound up, and my stream was getting tighter and tighter.

This much I knew: my bladder felt like a water balloon just ready to burst, and going to the bathroom was no picnic. At times I would only be able to evacuate just so much urine. That meant that I would have to make return trips to finish the job. That's not right, and I knew it. I also knew there was nothing familiar or normal about any of this. This became worrisome. Fear invaded what once were routine trips to the bathroom. Every time I knew I had to go I wondered. Every time I went, I knew. This was all too familiar a feeling, and I didn't like it one bit.

Soon it came time for one of my post-surgical hospital visits. This is when I would get to tell the doctor about what was going on. I was glad to be going to see him, but concerned, because I had no idea what he might say, or worse, suggest.

Each visit began the same. Clinic A always had its fill of patients. Time passed, or maybe not, and then it was my turn. By now I began to see familiar faces; nurses and receptionists also started to recognize me. I'm still not sure if it's good to be recognized. One of the nurses brought me back. I would be seeing her again over many visits. We talked, the normal questions were asked, and she did the normal reading of my blood pressure, weight, and concerns. They always ask about concerns or change. Here was my chance. So I told her about my concern, but it was weird to talk about it with her.

This is one more time where you have to talk to some total stranger about things you just don't share with anyone, let alone a woman you don't know. I thought I had gotten over all of that by now. Guess not. After making her notes on the computer she says, "It will be just a moment; the doctor will be right in." At least with the doctor I would be speaking man to man. That's a little better, isn't it?

Just as she said, it wasn't long before Dr. Frank walked in. We shared the typical niceties and introductions. Soon I discovered it would be time for Mr. Jelly Finger. No prostate, no physical exam, right? WRONG. Dr. Frank is old school; you check regardless. It wouldn't be this visit, but it would happen years later that I finally needed to know why he still did this exam if I didn't have a prostate. I asked one of doctors that I had met back when he was an intern during my surgery days. He said Dr. Frank believes that follow-up checks offer, in rare situations, an opportunity to detect things running a foul, things that would otherwise go undetected until they manifest themselves in different and more severe ways.

Makes sense, but it still gets old. Every time you go, and every time there's an intern or two Dr. Frank asks if they can take a turn. I don't remember any more how many times that's happened, or how many times I've heard, "That's how they learn." So you just smile, say OK, and bend over.

With all of the pleasantries behind us it was just the doc and I. "So how are you feeling?" he asked.

"Fine," I reply.

"Are you experiencing any problems?"

"Well" . . . I seem to have trouble saying what I need to say."

"Is everything going OK?"

So, I stumbled through telling the doc about the change in stream. It's not that it's difficult to understand; it's just awkward trying to describe how one goes about talking about such things. With that he called for a nurse. This was a deviation from the norm. That always gives one pause.

She arrived and he rattled off some medical jargon that I didn't understand. He also mentioned some size, which made no sense to me as well. Soon she returned with a short section of rubber hose, a section of catheter really. Then he asked me to take down my pants and lay face up on the table. Here we are, the doctor, nurse, and me, and I had to be the one on the table. Catheter and lubricating jelly in hand, the nurse stood to my left, and the doctor asks me to just relax. I had still not fully grasped what was coming next. Then Dr. Frank said, "Just try to relax."

Watching the doctor stand there I began to sweat a little more, and I couldn't help but watch the nurse or doctor's face for changes in expression, clues really, clues about our progress. See, I had a blockage forming. About an inch and a half or so up my urinary canal scar tissue was forming. At least that's how I understand it. Don't really know why. Nothing abnormal was ever explained, but there it was. The only way to correct this, or at least one way, is to take a smaller catheter and push it in past the part of the urinary canal that is affected. So taking the catheter in one hand and my, well you know, in the other he began to insert the tubing.

There I was in this kind of surreal experience. Again! I never saw this in any life plan I had ever envisioned. For the first inch it slid in easily. But then we hit what felt like a wall. So he grabbed hold harder and pushed more. With a little more effort it slid through. Once the catheter slid past that spot it moved easy again. The doctor moved the tube back and forth through that spot. Soon our visit was done. I thought, that wasn't great, but it wasn't bad either.

Boy, was I glad that was over. That concluded our visit for that day. Nice to end on a high. Out to the checkout counter I go. More niceties are exchanged. Discussions about more follow-up send you packing, new appointment dates set, new bottle of barium received along with a list of appropriate blood work. These blood tests are typically scheduled one week before the visit with the doctor so the results can be read and forwarded to the doctor. With a spring in my step and fresh bottle of barium in hand, I headed out. It will be three months before I'll get to visit Clinic A again.

At home things are better; the stream is better, bladder evacuation is better. Wow, I'm relieved. By now I have returned to work. Life is good. That whole other male thing still needs to be discussed, but for now, things seem dead in the water. But it's early and not unexpected at this point. We'll save that discussion for some later time. You and I are not quite as comfortable with each other yet. At least, I'm not. Sorry.

The weeks pass, and little by little things are returning to normal. Normal, as in the stream is narrowing again, and my bladder is full but emptying is again becoming an issue. In time I feel this time is worse than before. Yeah, great. That's all I can think about. I knew what they did the first time. I was no fool about what this might mean for my future. The first time was met with some fear of the unknown. This time was met with anxiety and fear—anxiety and fear of the known.

I thought about calling sooner, but three months isn't long, and anyway, I was hoping and praying it would correct itself. The appointment date arrived. Typically, I set my appointment times for the afternoon. That way I go to work for a half day till eleven, and then take half a day sick for the appointment. By now the stream was really narrow, almost needle like. Going was not pleasant. This scared me! There were times when I thought it might close off entirely. That would mean emergency surgery, as I saw it. The threat of that, even if it's in your head, is terrifying!

As I drove from work, a route very familiar by now, I could feel my blood pressure going up and up the closer I got to the hospital. It wasn't a perception; it was a tangible feeling in my body that my blood pressure was just going through the roof. In retrospect, it was a very interesting experience. And, no wonder, I knew what was coming. In the normal course of time I arrived at the hospital. I parked the car and walked into the cancer center with blood pressure still climbing. From the parking lot it is a short walk across the main drive that connects each building and up a small incline to the canopy that protects the entrance. They have valets to park your car for you if you like. For some, their health leaves them no other option. I am lucky to be walking in under my own power.

As I approached, the sliding doors part, just inside the lobby was a coffee cart, and then a station where security sits. The floors are tile, with some potted artificial plants. You go about thirty feet or so and then turn left. The first bay on the left is Clinic A. I picked out the velvet chair of my choosing after notifying the front desk of my arrival. Since one of the first things they ask you to do is pee, yet another sample, you can even get the small sealed cups right at the counter. I was in no hurry.

Soon my name was called. That old, but young, familiar nurse came through the door and called my name. I stood and signaled. She held the door as I passed. "Exam room. It's the third one on the left." By now I have seen enough of these rooms. The nurse takes my weight and height, and checks my blood pressure. You know when the nurse has to keep inflating that cuff higher and higher, well, you know it's going to be a doozie. I wish for the life of me I could recall the numbers.

How about one million over five hundred thousand? I don't recall her even telling me. She just said, "It's really high." I told her I knew it would be. I told her I could feel it just going up and up as I drove here. I told her I knew what was coming, and it's not good. She gave me a look like she somehow understood, and she said the doctor would be in soon and closed the door behind her.

There I sat; options and expectations swirled through my head. I like to be prepared for both. This was no different. In fact, it was worse. I needed to settle down. I needed to reinforce my resolve. Except who wants to run scenarios for this through their head? The swirling stopped only because there was a knock at the door. It opened, and in walked the doctor. What a relief.

The doc was friendly and very polite as always. "How are you doing?"

He always starts that way, but I feel like he really wants to know. Dr. Frank sits at the small table with computer and reviews the new nurse's notes. "So you're having trouble again."

"Yes," I say.

"How bad is it?" he asks.

"Well, I just can't go like I should. The steam is very narrow or tight."

"Can you tell me about how narrow?"

I've spent a lot of years doing woodworking, including a six-year stint in a custom cabinet shop. So it only seemed natural to describe it like the diameter of a nail. At the time it seemed like a good idea, but stupid in retrospect. So, I told Dr. Frank it was about the size of a small finish nail. Let's just say it was a very poor analogy.

He was unimpressed with my analogy, and commented on the nail, but I was serious. So I went on to explain how after our first experience dilating the urinary canal all was good for a while, but then little by little it began getting progressively worse. Once more he spoke to the nurse—I knew what was coming! The pictures our minds create are always available aren't they?

I reminded the doc that I had done a lot of walking when I had the catheter in, but he assured me this had nothing to do with my problem. He said, "We're going to try it again, and see how that works. Surgery of this nature really isn't an option that you want to explore." He again asked me to more lower my pants and get up on the table. So I hopped up on the table, pants at my knees, and that same nurse at my side. I could already read her eyes. Sad, squeamish, wincing-like—pick one. There she stood, at my side.

With gloves on, and catheter in hand, Dr. Frank began to push the tube up my urinary canal just like before, but not for long again. You didn't have to tell me. This time I could feel it more, and I could see it in the doctor's face. His brow furled and his eyes tightened; that thing just wasn't going anywhere. He asked the nurse to get a smaller size from wherever they keep those things. She left to return only moments later.

"Here we go again," he said. This time it felt like we were going to have better luck, until it hit the area that was causing me this problem. By now I could tell it was causing the doc even more concern. The nurse looked down at me with eyes that shared my pain, or at least what she could appreciate. He took a good hold and pushed like he was going through a brick wall. I groaned and groaned. My body stiffened. I wasn't going to scream, but no one would have blamed me. I clinched my fists and teeth. With the final push I cried out with my mouth closed and felt a pop! It had pushed through the blockage and moved up the canal freely. I exhaled in relief as my body relaxed on the table. When the doctor took out the tube it was followed a flow by blood. This time it was the nurse that groaned. Whatever was in the way, we TORE through it. I took a deep breath. The nurse grabbed some supplies and handed them to me to clean up the blood.

Wow, that was really something. That just raised the bar on my experiences with pain. Now it was time for instructions.

There's always aftercare. By the end of his instructions and my visit the doc handed me my very own take-home catheter. It was a short piece about six or eight inches in length just like the one he'd used, and a small tube of triple antibiotic ointment. The only way he said we could assure it would stay open while healing was for me to do it to myself at home. I was to use the catheter for as long as necessary, and as often as necessary, but trying to minimize the number of times per day, or number of times in a week.

That visit left me with a fear that if I waited too long I would be back on the exam table, or worse. So I'd go off to the bathroom and feed the tube up and down the canal, always with care, always with concern. But the only way to know if it was really healing OK was by not using it as frequently, and then trying it again. I hated this time. How long do you wait? How is it going to go? What if? This was quite possibly the worst part of all that I had been through. Demeaning, degrading, fear-producing—it wasn't fun anymore. I would stand in the bathroom and just pray, and hope, and wonder—was it going to go in easy? I hoped and prayed and wondered.

Early on I would catheterize myself every morning and evening. I'm no dummy. If there was bleeding there was a tear. If a tear, then a scab would have to form, which it did. In time pieces of the scab would be expelled during urination. This was a good thing. It was one less thing taking up space and freed up my stream even more. What a relief. Weeks later I would use it in the morning and then skip the evening. Then I tried a day or two, which helped my spirits a lot. After that, I went to almost a week, then a week, and finally stopped altogether. While this was great, inside I kept holding my breath. Time would tell.

You can rest easy. That was the last time I had to go through that. For many years I kept the catheter in the small surgical plastic bag in which they gave it to me. Finally, I threw the thing out. I'm not sure why I kept it for as long as I did.

Chapter 15

THE face of GRACE

The face of grace is profound in its appearance.

After a day filled with work, a run, and the demands of life, I love heading off to bed where I can just lie there for a while and watch the day's afterglow fade into the night's sky. I find it very peaceful. The struggles, elations, or humdrum of the day is washed away in the beauty of dark reds blending into deep blues and aqua greens. In their turn the stars begin to reveal themselves, hidden from earlier view, now revealed against the canvas of deep dark blue.

Tonight is one of those nights. The moon is almost full, glistening brightly with an iridescent silvery grey shimmer. These moments cause my body to shed the cares of life with deep sighs of relief. This night's sky carries with it wispy clouds set aglow as they pass by, pushed along by the invisible force we call wind. The moon's glorious in its appearance, restful in its comfort, bright with hope, as it illuminates the night's sky.

What has this to do with cancer, you may ask? By now, I have watched the moon for many a night. I watched as I looked up from my hospital bed ignorant of what lay ahead and during the days with the catheter. During those days, heading off to bed was the best part of the day. Or, as in the years that have followed, I ponder what now, or, what's next?

The moon is like a beacon in the night, the lesser of two luminaries that mark our sky. I love the moon because it reminds me of the constancies of life amidst a swirling mass of ever changing events, tests, appointments, surgeries, this date or that, this time or that, followed only by more tests, appointments, surgeries, dates, and times.

The light of the moon stands as a marker for the night, a marker that declares that the darkness will not prevail. Its light is the only thing that separates us from utter blackness. The moon is not always full, is it? It's not always that bright beacon in the night. Sometimes its light is only a sliver, like a tear in the black fabric of night. Other times a thick suffocating blanket of clouds attempts to hides it from our view.

Tonight, admiring the moon I am reminded. I am reminded that it is grace—and it IS grace. Grace in knowing that there are things in life that do remain the same. Grace that there are things in life we can count on, things in life that were set in motion before life began for me—for everyone.

As a part of who I am I love to encourage. So please, if only for a moment, let me be the moon. I want to shout to you who are trapped in the darkness of the night, "You are not alone!" As my window frames the night sky I have been encouraged to remember those who are out there looking up from their beds. But, we need to remember those even more who are unable look up, unable to find that light of grace that glows in the darkness and gives me peace.

I wish that in your times of darkness we could talk. I have discovered through times of hardship that God has blessed me with the gift of strength. I have more than enough to go around, and I don't mind sharing. Ask him, and he will give you strength. Ask him to give you a little of my strength. That's OK too.

I know that some of you don't believe, as I do, just who put the moon up there, and that too is OK. But, this much I know: many who don't pray or believe have been caught in the dilemma of what to do when the darkness rolls in like a thick black choking fog. All I can say is give it a shot. Ask. See what happens. And, if you feel better, give it another shot. What have you got to lose but the hold darkness has on you?

The moon has always been there, because that is its mission—to cross the blackness every night. Its constancy is on purpose, its presence a reminder—a reminder that we are being cared for, always. My hope is this: as the moonlight graces your window you find in it the light that will give light to your night and brightness to your darkness, as it does for me.

You are not alone. We share many more things than most of us realize. The moon's surface is a rocky, scarred sphere of highs and lows, darkness and light, shaped by meteors that once struck its surface. Helpless to defend itself from their attack, the moon is misshapen and yet beautiful, and each night it glows with the light of a greater light.

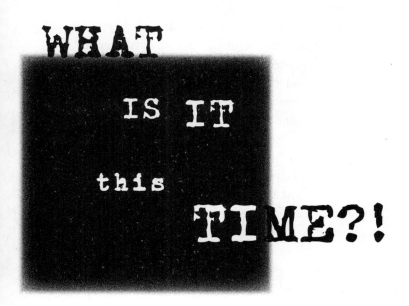

Chapter 16

WHAT IS IT this TIME?!

Another unexpected phone call
led to another unexpected
trip to the hospital.

With two surgeries behind me I was looking to the future and wondering what was next. But I never expected this. When many people go through a rough patch, it's not uncommon to look ahead with a degree of wonder, hoping it will be brighter rather than darker. By now I was rolling along. Then out of the blue the phone rings again, but this time it was a woman from Copley.

Now what? We talked for only a short time. I agreed and then hung up.

There I was back at Copley Hospital. This time dressed in black slacks, white shirt with a predominantly red tie with small dashes of black and white, and a salt and pepper sport coat. She had seen me roaming the halls during my chaplaincy internship and thought I would be the perfect candidate. During our short phone conversation she expressed how important it was that I feel comfortable, and I assured her I was glad to do it.

Because she and others knew me as one of their chaplains, and knew that I had just undergone both testicular and prostate surgery she asked if I would speak about my experience with prostate cancer. This was one type of program put on for Copley staff as part of continuing education and awareness. As part of my presentation I put together my personal facts and gathered some general statistics from the internet on prostate cancer and types of treatments. Most of the audience was female. OK, that was kind of weird, but a few guys showed up as well.

For forty-five minutes I gave them my story. You know, how I found out mostly by accident, depending on what you believe about life events. How I was not suspicious of any problems with my prostate, and how I didn't fit the typical model of someone with prostate cancer. As part of my presentation I addressed common signs associated with prostate cancer like difficulty with urination, or increased frequency with urination, stuff like that.

As I was nearing the end I felt it would be beneficial if I opened up the session for questions. I have never been afraid to disclose the details of my experience. So I said, "Does anyone have any questions? I'm not shy, and I won't be offended. Please ask me anything you would like—nothing is too personal."

The table in the conference room was long and narrow. Chairs filled with blank faces ringed the table. They weren't empty faces; they were faces that expressed those familiar feelings many of us experience during times like these. Your mind may be filled with questions. How should I react to what I have just been told? Was he really serious about his willingness to be open? How do I ask what's on my mind, especially when it's an uncomfortable subject for us to talk about?

After what seemed like hours rather than only a minute or two the silence was broken by a well-dressed man who had been sitting in on the program. "Everything you have described about symptoms sounds like me—urination issues, poor flow. I am experiencing all of these symptoms." I had also discussed as part of my presentation how prostate surgery usually causes impotency as a result of nerve damage. I talked openly about how I had been affected, and about the odds on having your erections return to normal. "But, I don't think I could ever have surgery if I needed it, because I would never want to end up impotent." He said that it was a big deal for him, and he didn't like the sound of that. You could tell that was going to be an issue should he be facing prostate cancer.

I commented, "When the rubber meets the road you have to be ready to make some choices, and this will be one of them."

Personally speaking, having an erection was never my measure of my manhood. There are many more things that I hope define me as a real man long before this one. I settled my score on this; you're on your own. I can't decide for you. As a matter of information, for you guys out there, in some cases the damage done during surgery leaves some impotent for the rest of their lives. This was not my experience, but it did take years for enough nerve healing to occur for things to return to normal, or almost normal. It should be rather obvious that with only one testicle and no prostate things wouldn't be normal again. I've never been fixed, but the prostate produces the fluid in which the sperm are carried. No prostate no fluid, and nerve damage does change the sensations and reaction time. Part of the aftercare from surgery includes a prescription for the little purple pill to help restore function. They give it to you for years.

There were a few more well-meaning questions that I can't remember. Then the man who spoke first blurted, "So what would you do if you were me?"

I didn't have to think. I didn't think. I just blurted back, "I'll tell you what I'd do. When you get out of this program I'd call your urologist if you have one and make an appointment as soon as possible." With that I asked if anyone had any more questions. They all just smiled.

The organizer and participants thanked me for coming, and I headed back to work. I couldn't help but wonder though if he was just going to go back to work? Was he going to interrupt work to make that phone call? How would I know? I just hoped he stopped whatever he was supposed to be doing after the seminar long enough to make the call.

I am currently employed by a municipality in their Public Works department. This is a very male dominated environment. And here, too, guys would come up to me after my surgeries and asked me about either one or both of my cancers. I was asked about how I knew I had testicular cancer, and how they might know. I was asked about prostate examinations and PSA testing. I was asked how either of those things had affected my life, and more importantly, my life with my wife.

Honestly, some men just grimaced and moved on. But others seemed to listen with genuine interest and wanted to know. As an insider to both of these cancers I found it interesting to watch how the different men reacted. Most of my conversations were done one-on-one, in places that gave us privacy and anonymity. Men are surely funny about these things. I think women are more open, but not being one I don't know for sure. It just seems like they are. We could learn to stop being so stubborn in the name of being macho. It might save a few men from suffering a lousy premature death, because they were too proud to find out before it was too late.

As part of my seminar I also touched on how testicular cancer very often moves up into the lungs and further if discovered too late, and prostate cancer moves into the bone. Funny, all either of them take to discover is a simple physical exam or a little blood test.

Beyond work I didn't advertise my cancers much, until this book project came to be. Most often I am approached through word of mouth. I have received phone calls from friends who know someone and wanted to know if I would talk with them. "I'd be glad too," is my usual response. Sometimes they call—most times they don't.

Sometimes when I think someone has questions they aren't sure how to ask, I leave bread crumbs. My invitations come in the form of short comments and allude to my confrontation with cancer. Or I talk about my rebuff of the survivor mentality associated with cancer. In times like these I make it known that I would be glad to share. Truthfully, as you may suspect, the audience means everything. Many men are cautious, afraid I will inform them of a symptom that will hit way too close to home. At the same time, they want to know, and are glad they can ask someone who was going to be candid, like it or not. My honesty has been a trait that has brought many to me for advice, or just to talk. I guess they feel safe.

Of course not every encounter works like this. Some men have avoided me like the plague, but eye contact and the walk off tell me a lot about what they would like to ask, but don't. Maybe they really don't want to know what's coming. Maybe they don't know how to talk about it themselves. Maybe they are uncomfortable, scared, and uncertain about how they would receive such news.

It's too bad. Silence might just be a first step down a path that will define, control, and consume you. Please, don't let it! Speak up. Ask the questions. Face facts head on, and don't waste time letting questions plague your mind without actually asking them.

Months later the grapevine gave me the news I had long wondered about. The man in the meeting had made the call. He got checked out. He found out that he, too, has prostate cancer.

This was one call I was grateful to have gotten—who would have ever dreamt! Mission accomplished. Nice!

Chapter 17

POSTER boy

**That's what the doc said to me:
You should be the Poster Boy for
prostate recovery.**

It's mid-August, time for another appointment, but this appointment was different. It was my one-year anniversary! Come to think of it, I never got a celebratory gift to mark the occasion. So much time together, and I forgot a gift.

This visit started just like all of the other visits I have described. The doc asked all of the usual questions and commented on how great I looked. I wonder if he doesn't say that to all his patients. By now we have a rapport. I always enjoy asking Dr. Frank how he is. This stuff can be so one sided. It's not like his life is free of the need for care, or crap, but we are often so self care focused we don't give our caregivers' lives a thought. So in an effort to level the playing field I try to ask him about how he's doing. It's not like we get into all kinds of disclosure, but at least I ask.

So here we are. We begin with the usual dropping of the pants with the assorted activities. He checks both incision scars, vitals, looks at the computer with my test results, and asks about how I am feeling generally. Then he asks me casually if I have any runs coming up. He knew I was a runner and asked if I had signed up for any races. So I told him I had signed up for the Chicago Marathon. He was surprised. Somehow in words I can't quote he told me that not many of his patients make such a phenomenal recovery in the first year. I thanked him for the complement verbally, but mentally passed it off as no big deal.

Much of my recovery had been a matter of hard work and trust. I knew what the rigors of training looked like. I had put many of these same rigors to work to get well. I have been *blessed* with a body that adapts and heals well. I have been *blessed* with strong mental toughness, at least most of the time. I have been *blessed* with a tenacious spirit to press ahead and believe. Training is hard work that includes a willingness to enjoy pain. Belief that I could do it, along with training supported by faith and prayer was all a part of my recovery program. I haven't seen the masses he has treated over the years, I was me, just being me. At least that's how I saw it.

MARATHON MAN

In time October finally arrived. It was time to run the 2005 Chicago Marathon. My finisher's time was 3:41:27. It was my best time to date. To non-runners this may not mean much. For some it will mean a lot. Usually, I'm not a big fan of going on about my running. Most times little is said, but it relates to the story, so I have chosen to tell you. It went according to plan; go out careful not to overdo it, and wait to see how the closing miles will go. That year I ran well through miles 22 and 23, walked about one block, ran again through the finish, 26.2 miles. My legs were sore and tired, but my mind was strong, and it was a good day.

This year (2010) I ran my worst time ever, and by a lot! You can look it up, but I'd rather not say. Time to train was complicated by health issues with my dad and then the death of my mom. Summer temps were abnormally high and race day temps were no exception. I also lacked the desire to do the long runs upon which success is built. None of this worked to my favor. But this just sounds like a lot of excuses.

This year's Chicago Marathon had 36,088 actual participants. Forty thousand signed up, but some don't show. The start time was 7:30 AM, but if you're running your day starts much earlier. Liz and Dan accompanied me this year. The morning's alarm went off at 4:30; we needed to be out of the house by 5:15. I wanted to be down there by 6:00ish. Inside my spirit gets antsy; I always like getting on the road. It's always better to be early than caught in traffic. I've learned that when you leave too late and get caught in traffic, antsy turns into frantic, frustrated, nervous, and surly.

I want to go into "present" mode again for a while as I describe the day. As we head down the toll road I wonder how many of the other motorists are running or are spectators today. As the skyline sharpens and the sun breaks the horizon we soon find out that most of the cars are carrying both participants and spectators. This year 1.5 million spectators would watch the race, many heading into the city just as early as we were. The highways act like funnels as everyone finds their way into the city and then looks for parking. I tend to park in the same place; it makes it simple.

Exiting the car, I check and recheck all the stuff I want with me. I evaluate the current temp, check my gear and decide what to wear, pack my gels (I take energy gels during the race as an energy supplement), put on my toe socks, and lace up my shoes. By now the sun begins to stretch across the city in a long stream of light. With it the temps and expectations begin to rise. Starting the race at about 45 degrees is great, but today's temperature is already 60 degrees. I just wanted the gun to go off. The sooner we get started, the sooner I will be done. Not exactly the best mental attitude on race day. The start is still an hour away.

Like salmon, we join the stream of spectators and runners. We move as one, pausing only for an occasional stoplight. The numbers grow. Today's the day. We make our way to the starting corrals. I start in Corral B because I have a seeded number, which means I had run a qualifying half marathon faster than 1:35:59.

By this point before the race you have walked through countless masses of humanity. There is a buzz in the air. Who couldn't help but get pumped up by now? I began to feel more positive. But, you work to keep your emotions in check; you don't want to waste energy on emotions. Rows and rows of potable toilets stand like silent sentinels, fulfilling their duty for the cause. Unless you've seen it, it is hard to imagine just how many there are. By now it is time to say good bye to Liz and Dan. They had their directions. They knew just where to go during the race to watch for me and where we would meet up when it was over. Liz gave me a kiss, I headed to Corral B, and they headed to the two-mile marker.

Dressed in a chartreuse tank top and black shorts, I entered the sea of humanity in Corral B. The total mass of people streams for blocks. If you've never seen it, it's truly a wonder. First, I sit, trying to stay cool inside. Thirty minutes pass. Then most of us begin to stand and pack together like sardines in a can; another thirty minutes pass slowly. Then the national anthem is sung, the wheelchair athletes are sent off, and now it's our turn. The gun goes off. Bodies press together and fight nicely for a space to run.

The early parts of any long race are occasions of checking in. I check in with my legs, taking stock of how they feel. I check my watch, monitoring my per mile splits. Go out too fast and die early; I know this first hand. It's also warmer than I prefer, and this too concerns me. I head out at eight minutes per mile. I had used a training time of seven minutes per mile, so now I just sit back and put my body on autopilot. The first half, 13.1 miles, is right on schedule, 1:45:00.

Time to take stock again. Actually, I do it all along the way, but I pay even more attention at the half way point. I'm thinking that the time is OK, but my legs just don't feel that spring that goes with a great run. There are those days when no matter what you ask of your legs they love to give it. I've been wondering if today would be one of those days. Now I begin to think it isn't. Oh well, only time and the miles will tell.

Everyone likes to talk about the 20-mile mark as the wall. I don't necessarily go along with that, but this year's wall came for me at mile 19. My legs seem to be out of gas. I am getting tired and frustrated. This is not the day I'd hoped for, trained for, or the race I came to run. I begin to do short stretches of walking, then run a mile, and then walk a block or so. By mile 23 the walks are getting longer, and the mile run in between is now a half mile. It really sucks when this happens. Times like these are when I recall my training runs on hot days, rainy days, and hard days, and you tell yourself you've done it before, so you can do it again.

I want to break 3:30:00. That isn't going to happen. Times like these make your head really begin to swirl. Quitting isn't an option but my legs are really sore and screaming back. They just ache. My whole body just feels tired and stiff, slow to respond when my mind tries to tell it something. My mind rages as I think about all of the 90 degree days I ran over the summer to get ready for this. My mind is frustrated with a race that started right on track, but soon derailed. I walk. I didn't come to walk. I watch others run past while I'm walking.

I pray for those I see being medically assisted along the way. At least that's not me, I tell myself. I don't mean to be arrogant. I just think it; human nature, I guess.

By miles 23 and 24 there is much more walking than running. Every mile seems longer than the next, but in time I click them off. In my head I tell myself all of the things I need to do to finish this. I remind myself I'm acquainted with all of these things, the mental race, the physical race because I've faced them before. At times I just tell myself to quit whining and tell my head to shut up. I hate my own weakness. Finally, I walk up the last hill and make the last left turn. The finish line is now one hundred yards away. I kick in a short burst. No one wants to walk it in. I run in, but not really. By now I wouldn't call what I am doing running. I can't wait to stop. Stopping at the finish line feels so good. I have never been so glad a race was over.

4:19:57. Yes, that was my time. I did all I could do that day, and it wasn't enough for me.

I walked, or should I say hobbled, through the finishers' corral and made my way through the masses, those who finished *ahead* of me, once more. Liz, Dan, and I chose a meet-up spot before the race and I couldn't wait to get there; I couldn't wait to see them. Thankfully, they came my way as I headed towards our meet up spot. When I saw them their smiles washed some of the soreness and disappointment away. There we were again, my family.

We headed back to the car but the walking was very slow. Muscle soreness and fatigue coupled with stiffness took any hope of skip out of my step. Sitting in the car felt even better. I shut my eyes for the ride home, another marathon in the books.

On the heels of my poorest marathon finish ever, I guess I've learn a few things in the past five years about life and cancer. It is not our best that can teach us the most about who we are, or what we are capable of. This "poster boy" ran slower, slogged longer, but grew more. Metal that is tested in expected conditions will never discover its true strength. But test it when it's really under pressure, and you'll know a lot more than before.

I had been using my training tactics on my cancer, a combination of mind, body, and spirit/Spirit. It's a lot like a marathon. I have set markers or goals that were used to gauge my progress or drive my progress. Motivation when running is huge, and motivators in recovery are also huge. I set expectations for my recovery and then worked to see them accomplished. I like to sign up for some special races early, and then keep my eye on them to motivate me during the grinds of training and various weather conditions. I don't stay home on bad days. Often I tell myself, "Look, you're out here and many are not." So I press on. If I quit now, it is even easier to quit later.

Some of my goals are realistic; others not so much. But, if you don't aim high what's the point? Anyone can be mediocre. I wanted, no, demanded of myself a stellar recovery, so I went after it.

Lessons. What to make of lessons? Well, I don't like that finishing time, and will tell you this is going to have to change. But, I don't know if I'll run another marathon, or do better if I do. We want to think we know. This year's finish doesn't make me feel much like a poster boy. I used to believe that if you train hard enough, or push yourself long enough, the outcome will be a good one. I don't believe that much anymore. Some days great training seems to mean little; conversely, I have been blessed with a good result despite my poor training. All this has taught me never to judge the efforts or energy of others, because you never really know what may be going on in their lives. In retrospect, I'm not sure what the doc saw that day. I'm not sure I know what a poster boy looks like.

Chapter 18

TIME HAS A WAY of changing YOUR THINKING

The passing of time so often affects us in profound ways that seem almost imperceptible on the surface.

Our spirits are changed; our thinking is changed. Had these years been cut short, much of what I have learned would have been derailed. These years have changed me, some to my benefit, others maybe not so much. What is of interest to me is how I have been changed, good or bad. Here are some of the ways my views of life have been changed.

CLINIC A

Clinic A is a place where I have spent an awful lot of time, much of it in the original red velvet chairs that adorned the waiting area. Short backed, nicely proportioned for a guy like me; rolled arm rests, short wooden legs, just the right amount of fuzzy—easy to sit in. These were the first chairs I sat in for many of the early years. Recently, in the last couple of years the hospital replaced them with a different style and color. I don't like them as much. I liked the red velvet chairs. By the time I came along they were a little dingy, a little worn.

At the beginning as I sat waiting I would bring a book and read. The other folks were stuck there just like I was. A waiting room for me is much like an elevator. We all face forward and no one talks. Bodies are there, but it feels empty. I may be interested getting to know others, but how do you start that conversation without coming off as weird? I didn't know how, and didn't think they'd want to talk anyway, so I brought a book to hide behind.

It's surprising how much time you spend waiting. Some days my wait time was nearly an hour if things had gotten off track. Some days that meant that my choice for reading left me hoping for more, so I closed the book, folded my hands in my lap, and minded my own business.

One time I recognized a teacher from my high school years. I'll bet he never saw me. I never had him as an instructor, but I'm sure it was him. He too found his way to one of those red velvet chairs, Clinic A, Loyola University Health System, *Cardinal Bernardin Cancer Center.*

Maybe this was the trigger, but I can't say for sure. I started looking at people's faces. I was bored with my book choice, so what else was I supposed to do? Our faces say a lot about us. I watched the young, especially the young. I felt bad for them. I wondered how I would feel if I were just a young kid rather than a 50-plus year-old man. I would watch the older gentlemen that fit the profile I didn't fit, accompanied by their wives, each taking their turn. Just like me.

You can learn a lot if you want to; it just depends on where you are placing your attention. That is, if you're looking at all. Some people might think it's none of my business. Some might even think it is an invasion of their privacy. As time passed I found myself looking at their faces less and less. You're probably thinking, that figures, it only makes sense. Sooner or later we can become desensitized to many things that should still stir our emotions. When this happens we're dead even though we live!

But, that's just the point. Imperceptibly to me a change was taking place. Over time I began to try to look into the person. I wanted a glimpse into what was really going on. I wanted to know more, see more deeply. So much of my previous care was done superficially, politely. Oh, don't get me wrong, I was operating in the sphere I knew, with the tools I had been taught. But my responses were devoid of the connection that helped me see others for who they were.

Sure, sometimes it's obvious. Hairless children in wheelchairs, men waiting at the counter receiving the same list of instructions I would soon be receiving. But this is only the surface. Until you can see in, you can't really see at all. So I asked God to let me see in. Have you ever asked to feel someone's pain, if only for a moment, so it touches you but does not crush you? Just a glimpse?

What I was taught by these chairs was that watching is not the same as looking. We can watch a lot of things without ever really looking at what we see. Looking is kind of like a camera. It helps us focus our attention in a particular direction in order to see.

Sadly, today's auto-focusing cameras rob the eye of details it would otherwise see. When they focus for us, many of our senses are derailed. Why? Because now we are not the one focusing; we're just letting the camera decide our focus for us, turning off our brain and perhaps even our emotional connection to the subject.

Older cameras demanded that we keep our eyes and brain in the game if pictures were to have a good result. These chairs helped shape my focus, and my watching was transformed into looking. These chairs were the place where my prayers would be shaped as I kept my heart in the game. Only to the degree that you can look inward are you truly able to pray for someone well. Did I get clear, sharp pictures? Sometimes.

One day when I returned to Clinic A for just another visit, I was saddened when I found the red velvet chairs were gone. I wish the hospital would have told me they were planning on getting rid of them, but of course they didn't. Why would they? I would have loved one of those older chairs. Just to take it home and remember. I can't imagine the number of stories those chairs could have told. I can't imagine the numbers of persons drawn to those red velvet chairs by no choice of their own.

The new chairs are what I am left with now. I have to get used to those chairs. After all, they're only chairs.

* * *

ON HOLD

"Mr. Beck, can you please hold?" I'm not alone on this; no one likes being put on hold. Today companies often add music, but that's just a diversion to keep us from being reminded that we have been set aside. We've all been there. Life is moving along, the phone rings, but before you can speak the person asks if they can put you on hold. That's annoying enough when it's just for a simple phone call—but what about when it's about your life! That's just how it felt when Dr. Frank said, you need to get a testicular ultrasound ASAP!

Just like that I wasn't going to work the next day. Instead, I was going to a hospital to get checked out! It doesn't take long before you are forced to make decisions about appointments, work, home, and more. Each of these things gets weighed, but the scales are set against you. Things you have thought to be important suddenly become almost irrelevant. We are pouring out our energy into living, and then they tell you, "You need to get this checked out." You see then just how quickly we jump through any and every hoop that is placed in our path.

By now I have had over six years of experience with these types of hoops. Sometimes the hoops seem to tighten like a strangle hold. Early on, this was lost to my thinking. Early on, I just wanted to be as compliant as possible. As time passed I began to recognize a shift in my consciousness. I began to grasp the hold that all of this stuff had on me, and everyone like me. We recognize that whatever this day may bring with it there is no place else you will be, or can be. I was saddened as I became touched by the large number of people who, like me, got their lives put on hold every day. I can't tell you how many times I have prayed for these folks. People like me, waiting like me, killing time like me.

Times like these happen more often than most of us would like to admit. But admitting it opens our consciousness to the fact that it might happen to us. So many mornings we head into our day innocently thinking we have the world by the tail. What a joke!

When Liz read this section she asked, "Is this really how you see life?"

I assured her I did, and said, "Tragedy is always no more than a second away. That's how I see it."

She replied, "That's really a morbid way to see life."

"Maybe, but I don't see it as morbid. I see it as being prepared. That's all, just prepared." Funny thing is, I told Deb, a running friend of mine, this same statement, and she too thought it was "morbid," using that exact same word Liz used. I'll leave it up to you to decide which perspective is right.

Think about it, who puts a date for cancer into their PDA, or on their calendar? Tell me how much control you believe you have. If we want to be honest, do we really know what the next second will bring, or what about the next day, or week, or year? We do plan, don't we? Our next vacation or, for me, my next race. Which of us hasn't known or heard about someone who died suddenly? The news never gives us break from the suddenness of life. No notice. No warning of any kind. I'm not trying to be flip, but it's true, and I do feel bad for their family and friends. Futures full of plans, and BAM! Tragedy or destiny strikes.

I like putting events or things out there in my future. Hopes, dreams, or things I would like to do, or see. When it comes to my running I have planned for some races eight months in advance, especially when it's a marathon. I like putting runs on the horizon; they give me something to shoot for, train for, and dream for. I like the way they can carry me past or through times that are less friendly to my spirit. Not being a fan of winter much anymore I like to look forward to a fun spring race. I like markers; they remind me I have days yet to live. Make me believe I still have some control. Whether I actually make it to those markers is not up to me.

We plan, and plans fall through. We make appointments, and they too fall through. Life, the meaning of life, our purpose and goals, power and weakness, each has a tenuous hold on a reality that can shift like the sand or change in a moment.

Funny that we hold time like it belongs to us. When "my life" has been put on hold, at times I begin to think a different standard of measurement is being used to mark time. There have been days when it seems I was caught between two worlds at war. A war where decisions I am not a part of will determine just how many days I may have left.

* * *

CHORES

Liz and I divide up the work around the house. Yard work is mostly mine, but that doesn't stop her from cutting the grass if I'm tied up with a larger project. We have always found ways to pitch in and work alongside one another to get things done. Each week we both have our list of inside work as well. I do the laundry much of the time, a task that started back when I was in school. A small office that I used for studying is in the lower level of our home. Right next to this office is the laundry room, which makes it easy for me to keep track of when the washer or dryer needs attention.

Along with the laundry I often find time to vacuum. Liz tackles other jobs, such as the bathrooms, which I am not afraid to do when necessity calls. Typically, Liz washes the floors and we both flip a coin, though not really, for dusting. I think dusting is my least favorite. Liz isn't a knick-knack freak, but that doesn't mean there isn't a lot of stuff to move in order to dust. That's especially true in the bedroom, where we have the most stuff to move between each of our dressers and night tables.

Come to think of it, I suppose my night table may not be so different from yours. On our night tables we have the phone and answering machine, two pictures, and a book. I try to read a book most often just before bed. It happens to be a cherry colonial nightstand with a dark reddish burgundy stain. Its one drawer with two handles is cluttered with phone numbers, a small flashlight, and other random stuff that just seems to find its way into a drawer.

I also have two pictures on my night table. One of the pictures is a silhouette of a runner against the horizon at dusk. My son gave it to me when he was about eight or nine. At the top of the photo in large italic print are two words—*The Goal*. At the bottom it reads, "Forgetting what is behind and training toward what is ahead, I press on toward the goal to win the prize for which God has called me heavenward in Christ Jesus." Philippians 3:13-14

The other picture is of my wife Liz and me. It's in one of those wood frames that folds in half with a place for a picture on one side and a saying on the other. We got it as a wedding gift. The picture frame half, of course, holds a picture from our wedding day. Liz is in her bridal gown, and I'm in my tux; both of us wear bright smiles full of promise—we were much younger then. The other half of the wooden folding frame has the words, "The two shall become one" . . . Matthew 19:6. Joined in marriage. Joined in this world of cancer. My cancer has become her cancer of sorts. What irony!

The nightstand also has a lower shelf as well. I don't put much on that shelf. Only two things sit on that shelf: my bottle of barium and the instructions for taking the barium on a printout from the hospital where I have the paperwork needed for my next appointment. Early on those bottles moved on and off the shelf quickly. Three months—time to go! Then they stayed for six months, and eventually a year. In the meantime, I dust around it like any other object.

They never warned me that some side effects take years before they begin to show up. Most of these don't last long; they manifest themselves in different forms, or at different times. I wonder if the medical community even understands they exist?

Chapter 19

Life and LIVING, death and DYING

Each day we all make choices about how we will spend our time.

In our home Liz uses a monthly calendar it to keep up on all of our upcoming appointments, dates with friends, special events like birthdays or anniversaries. Important stuff. Stuff we want and need to remember; the *good* stuff. But, who pencils in the *upcoming* days lost to illness, accident, or disease when we do not even see them coming? What if we were given a calendar that would highlight those days?

Today we have so many different devices to measure or mark time that it is mind-boggling. Our pace has become so fast. Here in the Midwestern suburbia it seems many times it is almost impossible to keep up with time itself. Especially on those days when I found myself waiting and waiting, I felt like I could see the minutes of my life running out before my very eyes. Like sand pouring through an hourglass, my life was being poured out. Some days I could almost see a pile of sand accumulating at my feet right there in the waiting room. I pictured each of the other patients, family, or friends there that day, each with their piles of sand—some barely ankle deep, some knee deep and growing. Some I imagined I could no longer see. Those were suffocating!

When we're young we walk around with that carefree feeling that our whole lives are ahead of us. With plenty of time on our side our minutes loom large. I never thought much about my minutes. I didn't, at least not until so many of them were being consumed by all this cancer junk. Minutes were like grains of sand emptying hopelessly away never to return. Doctors' appointments, tests, surgeries—all like sand draining out, whether I liked it or not. No way to stop them. No grip strong enough, no way to refuse what you are never asked. Just gone!

So one day, just for kicks, I began to calculate my minutes. I added up the hours of my appointments, which by now have filled more than one day. One day equals 1440 minutes, by the way. My surgeries consumed four days, and my testing has also consumed days. That's at least a week. One lost week equals 10,080 minutes. When we lose one year we lose 524,160 minutes! Statistics tell us there are 28 MILLION people affected by cancer. If each of us lost only one minute, that is equivalent to 53.4 YEARS! When you stop and consider that it is not hard to lose one year, that's 28 million years of living lost to this disease! Wow!

But cancer never happens in a vacuum. My wife Liz and son Dan, two living parents (at the time), four close family members, and a dozen or so close friends all were in this with me. That equals 21 other people who spent some amount of time out of their lives thinking, praying, or worrying about me and my situation with cancer. By the way, I think this number of 21 loved ones and close friends is a conservative estimate. If you multiply that number times 28 million cancer patients you have 588 million lives affected by cancer. Unfathomable! But, that's not where the real theft of time occurs.

The real stealers of our time are some of our closest friends—Fear, Worry Anxiety, Hopelessness, or Control. These vile attackers are rooted deep within the world of cancer. They are the true robbers. I was robbed of time during these events like doctor's visits, sure, but were they the real threat to my life's minutes? THEY WERE NOT! These insidious foes are the ones you need to face if you want to win in the arena of saving time. It doesn't mean your cancer will go away or that you will gain any lost time back. What it does mean is that the time you have you will spend in a better place.

I never really kept a total of how much of time I've lost. I haven't given much thought to what I might have done with those lost days or weeks, or even years. I'm not saying I can't think of better ways to have spent that time, but I wouldn't change how they were used either.

So, that raises some very good questions about life—about living and death and dying. About control, and who has it. When I stop and consider how many things were going on inside me the number swells even more. Beyond the cancers that had been growing inside me I was growing in ways I never imagined. Inward changes were taking place, some already mentioned. I don't think there is a person alive who hasn't wondered at some point about their own existence, or death, or dying—the real nitty-gritty. I believe it's only natural to do so. Oh, for a while we may live what on the surface seems to be these invincible lives, but one day, sometimes in a flash or in a split second, mortality rears its ugly head, and now what is a person supposed to do? My "Bam!" moment made me ask: What would I believe—believe about me, about life, about death, about cancer? About my identity?

So, here's some of what I believe. I believe I was knit together in my mother's womb by God. This has enabled me to trust God that this struggle with cancer too is part of his divine plan, instead of blaming God. What I'm not is some random hanging file folder. I am not a test result. I am not adrift. I'm not a victim! I am not a casual observer; I'm a player, and this is my stage. We each have a life's stage. Our opening curtain is called birth, and it is followed by acts like these depicted in my story. My acts make up one man's journey with life, faith, and cancer, one day to be followed by a closing curtain. Does it bother you to see your life in such simple construction?

It doesn't bother me. I have come to a place that will let me say what for most of you may come as an impossible statement: *Cancer doesn't shorten lives.* Oh, I know we keep hearing statements like, "They lost their battle with cancer." But, I won't die prematurely from cancer, but cancer may bring my life to an end. The number of the days of my life is what they are; I will die no sooner than I am to die, and cancer cannot change that. Oh, it may be the means by which my appointed number of days find their conclusion, as I just said, but I don't believe that so much as one minute, one second, of my life can be made shorter by cancer. My life's power is not held in cancer's hand; it is held in the hand of Another. This is what I believe. When you die from cancer and still have managed to retain your identity—you haven't lost—you've WON! "They lost their battle" is yet another term that's GOT to go!

Let's face it. A construction worker falls forty stories while clinging to a sheet of plywood and survives. Sky divers land in softened farm fields when their chutes don't open, and live.

There is one unavoidable truth: it is appointed for us to die. Appointed like an appointment—the time, the place, the way. I met death once; he made a house call. Maybe that's why I don't fear death like most.

Truth be told, we hear about people every day who head off into a day full of promise, full of plans, places to go, people to see, work to do—and bam! They're killed on the way to work or become a victim of some random crime. In some cases what seems to be an insignificant event suddenly brings about a death we never saw coming.

My mother's death was like this. We were worried about my dad, but Mom, she was going to live forever. If she were here she would tell you. Then suddenly, one day things changed, and five days later she passed away. As part of my eulogy, I told all in attendance, "There was no one more surprised by my Mom's death than her." And that was the truth. See, we just never know. And yet, many choose to ignore the obvious—our days are numbered, and death only comes when it's our turn to go.

I believe we get one shot at life. Cancer has not shortened my life, but it has shaped it; or has it, if it was always meant to be this way? Can you find peace where you are that will let you embrace the events of your life? Can you be comfortable there? It hints at our relationship with Control. Are you close? Are you a slave?

Once I gave up control, other unwelcomed emotions attached with that found out quickly they weren't welcome here either. I'm sure those who know me best would tell you I still like being in control, and I do like to feel I have some power or control over the basic life decisions I make. But, I know this thinking too may be a myth. Here I'm just trying to find the words to impart some wisdom that taught me not to fear death or attempt to control my own end—because we can't. I don't have any idea how my future will play out, but one of the things I learned from my Momma was that I wasn't about to waste any more time than necessary on cancer. Mom loved life, and she knew cancer first hand.

Sometimes we let things control us that we know are no good for us, but we do it anyway. I'm here to say, YOU can choose to get rid of some longtime "friends" that just aren't worth keeping around anymore. Please, tell Control and his buddies Fear, Anxiety, and Worry to take a hike, and see what happens next.

I know that sounds wonderful and nice. I can hear it now, "Sure that's easy for you to say." But it's not. And it's not for me either. Admittedly, I fought for Control and faced Fear. Have I been anxious? Absolutely! And if there's one enemy I have yet to address, it is Anger.

Anger really pisses me off. I don't like getting angry, and cancer never made me angry. What angers me is that time loss. Oh, not the scheduled ones. I know they're coming, so that's OK. What I'm talking about are those days when you think you have everything accounted for, and then the flood gates open. All it takes is one phone call, and every plan you had goes right out the window. This makes me angry! These times make me burn inside! In these moments my head spins with all of the stuff I was planning on doing, none of which is going to get done, and it makes me angry. Time has become such a valuable commodity to me. Some days, life seems so short. How is anyone supposed to know which parts of life are times well spent when blessing takes the shape of a dreaded disease, and real life is found in the threat of death?

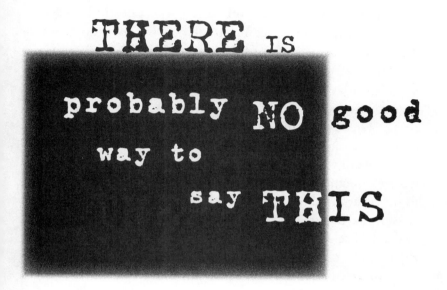

Chapter 20

THERE IS probably NO good way to say THIS

For many of you who will read this book, there may never be a good time to have this conversation.

But, it is one we must have, and now is as good a time as any. Some of you may even feel attacked—that is not my intent. Please believe me when I say that. I hope you can by now. Earlier, I alluded to what I call "survivor syndrome." The use of the term "survivor" is something I never liked much, so I just ignored it. I just wanted to be me, but it seemed everywhere I went this term kept popping up, causing a disquieting feeling in the pit of my spirit. Please let me explain.

I am not a survivor! I am just Guy in the act of living. Not a person trying to stave off death—I met death! It's kind of both funny and infuriating to me how we allow events to define us for the rest of our life.

About three years after my cancer surgeries I was attending a Saturday night church service. What I didn't know was that it was some kind of cancer awareness month or something. "Great," I thought as they highlighted this at the beginning of the service.

Generally, we walk in to a worship service kind of like we do a doctor's office and scan the setup. Where do I want to sit? Your mind is at work deciding if you need to be by an exit, or maybe down front—funny how those seats are always available. I selected something about half-way back, just to the right of the center. The church had an auditorium-style set up, individual seats that folded up just like at the movies. No drink holders though.

Soon the service started. It opened with the usual contemporary songs for this type of church. The passages were read, but I can't remember them anymore. I don't remember the sermon either, for that matter. Then there was a break in the service. The pastor stood up front and asked, "Is there anyone out there who has had, or currently has, cancer? We would like to pray for you." I looked around at those who were raising their hands. My brother and my niece Christine were with me, and they both looked over at me. I just turned and looked back. There wasn't a chance I was raising my hand!

It was then that something began to grow inside me. It was a feeling of annoyance and a kind of inner anger. More raised their hands, the people bowed their heads, the pastor led his prayer. We soon continued on with the service, and shortly after it ended—but not for me. That fact that I couldn't shake what had happened in the service annoyed the crap out of me. In many ways that night gave birth to my anti-survivor mentality and my resentment of the "survivor" term, a term that has probably single handedly given birth to the apparently *welcomed* survivor mindset. All I kept thinking about the rest of that service and beyond was all of the other people who could have really used some genuine, heartfelt prayer that night, but we didn't pray for them. We didn't even ask, "How can we pray for you?" We didn't ask, "What help might you need?" "What challenges are you facing?" "What other type of mental, physical, family, or personal struggles are at war within you right now?" I know without knowing, if you know what I mean, that many others that night were in a lot worse shape than I. They may have been barely hanging on, wanting the help I was offered, but they didn't get it.

It is that picture—that mental picture—that still fuels the fire of disgust and disdain I hold within even to this day. I can still remember how it felt. I can still see it in my mind. It still conjures up the same frustrations and anger. If only I would have been strong enough to stand up and tell every one of them, "Listen, we need to stop painting cancer patients like they're a special needy group. We are not special! I'm not needy! Maybe some of us need to get over this kind of thinking, and remember that many others have it even worse! I can almost guarantee that right now examples of things even worse are racing across our brains as you run through a list of possible diseases no one ever wants to face.

Please don't be put off. I know that there are a lot of cancer folk who use the term "survivor" as part of their everyday vocabulary and recovery, often with a sense of pride. But, this never worked for me, or for others I have spoken with. Once I spoke to a gentleman who described his wife to me as a double survivor when he learned that I, too, had two different cancers. He didn't know I really had three—add skin cancer to the list. With this gentleman what struck me was the fact that we had only just met, and I didn't really know him or his wife.

It wasn't that I wasn't sympathetic towards them both. I really liked the guy, and I'm sure his wife is an awesome woman. But it just bugged me that this was the first thing he told me about her.

Another time the same thing happened at a church picnic. I was introduced to a lovely woman who, before she even told me her name, described her whole battle with cancer. I wanted to know her name, but it seemed rude to interrupt. I kept thinking in my head, "Tell me about you—who you are, what your name is. Not this! You must be so much more than this disease!" But the disease had overshadowed her real identity, and it made me sad.

What concerns me is that our culture is creating a whole new disease I call "survivor syndrome." And we don't even know it! Is there any other disease on the planet that carries with it the badge of survivor? Every day many diseases take lives, ruin families, and rob the living of their dignity! We are not alone when it comes to lives being ripped to shreds. I just wish we would stop calling ourselves *survivor*.

Let's face it, there are a lot of terms that surround cancer. I also greatly dislike the term "remission." I bring it up because our "survivorship" is often linked with this term. I looked up the definition just for kicks. This is what the dictionary said about the term remission: "a temporary or permanent decrease or subsidence of manifestations of a disease." Well, if that doesn't want to make me jump on board, nothing does! "Temporary or permanent decrease or subsidence." So, which is it, temporary or permanent? Sounds to me like a term you might use when you're trying to hedge on a bet.

I'm not trying to be mean, though it may sound that way to some. My point is this: why exchange one label for another? Stop labeling the terms of my disease with other terms that carry with them all kinds of other junk! How about, "Guy, right now we see cancer." Or, "Mr. Beck we don't see cancer at this time." Period. No hedging, no promises, just the facts as they are today. I'll prefer to let tomorrow worry about tomorrow, thank you very much. I'm also smart enough, as we all are, to know that when we are told cancer is gone today, no one can offer guarantees about anyone's long term future. For some, the positive prognosis they are given stands the test of time. What a blessing that is. But for others, the good prognosis will not be correct. Unfortunately, it has been my experience that regardless of what I have been told about my future, this news cannot prevent questions and wondering from pervading my thoughts no matter how may years it has been. I plan on wondering for the rest of my life.

When you're labeled with cancer it becomes your identity. When you're labeled with survivor you're a hero barely hanging on. *Survivor syndrome*—my term—is not medically recognized, but it keeps us in a never-forgetting web of control. You cannot be truly free unless you reject all labels and remain true to who you are. Labels keep us and everyone else from seeing the real us. It's as if these labels were literally stuck on our bodies for visible display.

Another fear I have is that you may be hiding behind these terms, or worse, enslaved to them. I hope not. My plea, my cry is this: "BE YOU!" You don't need to be afraid to let the world see you for who you really are. I realized that I am not defined by cancer. By shedding labels of any kind, I can live life as Guy and be Guy, wherever the journey ahead leads.

In my case, survivor was called, "watchful waiting." You remember, from back at the beginning of my story. Oh, they didn't say it that way or remind me at each visit, but what was "watchful waiting" supposed to tell me? Who watches and waits when they know nothing is going to happen? Tell me? People don't stand in line, sometimes for days, for nothing. We don't slow our cars through an accident scene because we're really concerned about safety—we want to see blood, like sharks in the water. We watch, stretching our necks, and sometimes causing another accident in the process. The people who wait, they wait because they know something is suppose to happen next—like Black Friday specials the day after Thanksgiving.

My dad is a "Vet." Second World War, South Pacific, and he's proud of it. That term, "vet," got me thinking. You know, I kind of like that term "vet," if I had to pick one. Cancer in many ways is much more like a war than some odd event that suddenly tries to take your life. In war we have skirmishes, or small, medium or larger battles. At other times we convene a war strategy in the war room. Think about it. Hospitals and clinics with conference rooms or exam rooms are like war rooms where we map out our strategies and plans of attack. Then we choose a day similar to a planned invasion and get the troops ready—doctors, nurses, specialty staff, family members and friends, even clergy—each with their marching orders. We use special weapons, special ammunition, and special uniforms. How interesting!

Similar to war times, some enlist while others are drafted, like it or not. I was drafted and I didn't even know I was being drafted. Then, once I noticed "my notice" I tried to evade the draft by ignoring my notice (when I physically knew I had a testicular issue). The battle had begun long before I was willing to recognize it.

BONDS OR BONDAGE

This is another thing, something I would term as corporate solidarity, where bonds are forged in the fires of wins and losses. I'm not much of a joiner, but I long to be a part of the cause. If you can't tell by now, I struggle with joining because joining seems only to reinforce this social pressure surrounding the *cancer craze*. Cancer brings unlikely people together just like war. Battle stories are shared. Years of service are shared. Conversations identify friends or family, sons or daughters, moms and dads. We have our walking wounded, or our causalities. There are battle scars; I have two. As in war, when you come back, you're celebrated, or should be. When you don't come back, you're mourned and your life is celebrated, or should be. The cancer war has days marked by joys and defeats. This war also leaves many with lifelong pain and families confronted by a new face to life. Bodies may be irreversibly changed. What choice did they have?

So what term would I pick to define the person who goes through the battles, if it were up to me? After spending probably what has been way too much time mulling and thinking, questioning and tossing terms back and forth in my brain, I could only come up with one: How about Guy, or Frank, Mary or Joan—how about that? How about leaving us with nothing less than our names? How about that!

Freedom is no freedom at all if it is not absolute. Even memories have the power to enslave, and *survivor* is just another term that enslaves if by its very use we are not freed from the power of those memories.

So, rather than beat this to death, I'll just stop here. That's kind of all I wish to say about that anyway. So, PLEASE don't call me a "survivor." Don't perpetuate the syndrome. Because being free from all labels allows me to be FREE to be Guy!

Chapter 21

WHO do YOU think you ARE?

So, after all this, who am I?

That always makes for an interesting question. In retrospect it seems I have been working to sort out this question and my experience with cancer for a long time. Each of my days, my life events, have all become a part of the process. Wisdom born in the fire has taught me an important truth. Ignore who you really are, and well, good luck with that.

Ironically, most of us either haven't done the hard introspective work it takes to "really" discover who we are and then come to terms with that person, or we simply don't like what we see when we begin to look, so we create elaborate ways to hide, followed by pretending we like the "new" us.

In an atmosphere of disclosure I admit without hesitation that I was not always this spiritual guy walking around all full of confidence. In my very early days, I didn't care much about church and God. Oh, I went to church because my mom "dragged" us. In retrospect, I guess the principles were always there to guide me, but I didn't understand. It's not as if I was openly against God, but it's not like I thought church had much to offer either.

During my earlier adult years I did a lot of hiding. I used to hide behind an ever-changing facade. If people can't put their finger on just who you are, or if you're just one of those filler people no one really notices, you're safe. If people don't see you even when you're there, or they can't define you, they can't hurt you. It's not unlike sitting in the back row or taking a back seat when others are around. For me, moving in the periphery was safer. So, I would participate in only selected things, and was not a joiner. But, because I wasn't one who had to follow the crowd it also helped keep me out of trouble. I simply went to work or school and then back home.

My brother and I were close, and we had only a few close friends. Group events were just not our thing. While I participated in high school gymnastics with a passion, I never attended other school functions or games, no proms, no graduation. Even the parties tied directly to the gymnastics team went unattended. I recall being asked one last time by a young lady associated with the team whose name was Terry. It was our senior year, the last home meet. Gary (my brother) and I were walking down the hall after the meet. She stopped us and said to the best of my recollection, "You guys haven't come to one party in four years. Would you like to come to this one? It's the last one."

As vividly as if it was yesterday I can still hear my answer, "Well, we haven't come to one yet, so why start now?" I didn't see the value or point. I was comfortable in seclusion. More likely, I felt safe. Gary and I were liked, and we liked our teammates, at least most of them. I'm sure Terry felt some degree of hurt or frustration or anger. Now, I wonder why she even tried. It had been four years. I wouldn't have asked me after all that, if I were her. Today, if given the chance I would like to apologize. She never deserved my abrupt and rude response.

Truth be told, I just wasn't much for the social scene. Introspection tells me I was socially immature. Perhaps Gary and I had too many years of being joined at the hip as identical twins. But we enjoyed it then and thought nothing of it.

Another rationale I used on myself back then was this: if I don't let anyone see the real me, it can't be used by them against me. When they couldn't get a fix on me it kept me in control. It's not that I would go to great lengths to change who I was; I just never made it real clear, and I would change up little details from time to time. Then, when someone would get to me I just wouldn't show it. Good or bad, I kept them guessing by never offering any real exposure. I felt it served me well at the time.

Over time this kind of running got old, or finally, I grew up. That's probably the best way to put it. I didn't like hiding, or circling around, or living with the person I'd created. That was very tiring. Instead, I wanted to be the guy who felt comfortable with Guy. So much of life is really a process, isn't it? So, little by little, I began not to care in a good way. Not care what others might think. I would have described myself as shy, and I would blame a lot of it on being an identical twin. For as long as I can remember, Gary and I were always the "twins." We didn't even need names. Most everyone got them switched around anyway. Gary would answer to Guy. I would answer to Gary. It was just easier.

If there was one thing that has bothered me about being an identical twin, it was my loss of identity. By now you should know that identity with me is huge. Much of this book is about identity. It started way back then, and I didn't even know it. I wanted to be me, and have people know me for me. I'd spent too many years being defined as "one of the twins." Then I slowly allowed myself to be who I really was. Does anyone calculate what all these things cost us, or how hard it is to become who we are really meant to be?

In time I would meet Liz, my wife to be. Do you know what it feels like when you meet someone who grants you total freedom to be you? They like YOU! Oh, I know that while dating we try to put on all those facades, but one day when the shade is raised and the light of day shines in, well, we can't hide what we really look like, can we?

Over the years, Liz has put up with a lot. I told her from the beginning, "I can't say for sure where life will take us, but I promise you it will always be an adventure." As Liz told you earlier, I've been faithful to that. Thanks to Liz's love for me, this Guy no longer felt threatened by being who he was. What you see is what you get. This is who I am. Liked or disliked, I am who I am. When I understood this, it made much of life a whole lot easier. The only mold I needed to fit into was the one God and I saw for me.

Another part of who I have become has to do with running mental scenarios through my head. I like mental gymnastics, as my high school science teacher called it. My brain is always running, even when I'm not. Stuff is always going around in there. I'm always thinking of two or three things at a time. Sometimes I wish I could turn it off, but, oh well, it's my brain and I'm stuck with it.

My approach to cancer wasn't any different. I would take the events as they would come and run outcomes in my head. I would run doctor visits, tests, or even the surgeries with their results and recovery in my head. Good, bad, or something in between, this helped prepare me for what the real outcome was to be. I tried to see them. I tried to see myself, like those out-of-body experiences you hear about. See myself walking through an appointment or recovering from testing or surgery, as I said. Because I had already worked it through in my head the reality seemed only a natural transition. No surprises.

As a downside, it also has flattened out my overall spectrum of emotions. What do I mean by that? By choosing to keep everything on an even plain I am protected from extremes. We all like the ups but wish to avoid the downs. When confronted with a down you can level it out by minimizing the ups. I see good results and bad as a matter of fact rather than good or bad, and then I just move on. Results are results; they don't have emotions of their own. We attach emotion. I try to cut emotion out of it. We are free to do this, should we choose too, but it don't mean that all areas of life need be emotionally void—that would be just plain stupid.

When Liz asks how an appointment went, and she finds out everything is OK, she's excited. You can see it physically on her person. I don't share the same elation, but I also don't spend lots of time worrying when a result is less than ideal. In these settings I prefer to replace emotion with attitude. I always have an elevated level of attitude. I pride myself, good or bad, on attitude. Attitude, as I see it, is not an emotion— it is a state of mind. Attitudes, the things we say or think, plant seeds. Wheat or weeds, nutritious or noxious, every day we make choices about how we will respond to our treatments, or how our loved ones can influence those they love. Attitude is huge! Someone close says, "Oh, you'll never . . . ," and the words fall like stones against our flesh. Tell me what I can't do—please. Please tell me! Negative words used to be like food to me; please fatten me up and see what you get. But, that was before I didn't care what you have to say. Once I became comfortable with me, what people had to say became powerless over me.

Many don't even know they are stoning us by simple words or looks that tell us, "You're not looking so good." Or, "This treatment or recovery is going to be tough, and I'm not sure how you're going to come through it." Others, the smarter ones, offer their energy and hope and tell us, "I'm sure you'll bounce back fast." Encouraged, we press more, fight harder, and take steps lifted by the invisible power that encouragement brings to attitude. Tell me what I can do—please. Please tell me!

One day it may be you who faces cancer. Or, maybe you already are. But, I hope not. This much I know: thanks to what began in those earlier years, strengthened through Liz's love for Guy and rooted by faith and a call to "make it a mission field," my attitude was and is set. I must move forward. I cannot go back. It took a long time to get here. It took a long time to find out who I was, who I am meant to be. Cancer came along and tried to redefine me. Not now. Not after all that work. The real irony came when cancer found out that it helped make me even more who I was, not who it tried to make me become. Take that!

Just so you know, in an air of openness I've never done the crash and burn. I can't. I won't let that happen. I'm digging in my heels on this one. Maybe I haven't been really pushed or tested yet. Time will tell. But, this much I know: My attitude is not rooted in some hoped for vague vision of a better day or in trying to bring about some personally concocted dream. It is rooted in something far greater than that. When the winds of challenge come, it won't take long for everyone to see just how deep your roots are. Your attitude must be rooted in something greater than yourself, or your bad days will be really dark.

There are those days, because they come, when I might just go ahead and lie to myself. I tell myself exactly how I am going to bounce back, one hundred percent, no ifs, ands, or buts. It usually helps for a while, proving a short-term break from reality, and that's OK too. Some days a short break is all anyone needs. Some days I'm just a guy trying to hold it all together—my way.

Since you and I know that lying to ourselves isn't the best solution, may I suggest adding some layers of protection against lying? These protective layers have helped me against the dark times, or having to lie about what's really going on. These layers can come in many forms. For example, I found positive comments about recovery to be helpful. I have fed off of negative energy, but it's not healthy. We are what we ingest. When you're told that you're looking good, or that your recovery is moving along better than expected, and you know they are being truthful these honest words lift your spirit. When addressing those facing difficulty, if you can't be positive, then just shut up. Instead of telling someone it will be long and hard tell that person you know they have the stuff to get through it. More harm can be done than you will ever know. And because we all walk through this differently, and all suffer, this may be your true feelings and they are valid, but it's just not helpful when verbalized in front of the patient. More than likely, they will never tell you how your words hit them like stones upon their spirit.

Faith is a great attitude lifter. As often as you can, meet with friends you trust who are strong prayer warriors or gifted at encouragement. Allow yourself to rest in their comfort. There is peace to be found in close faith-filled friends. This can come in the form of conversations you might have with them. Having someone in your life who allows you to vent or express uncertainties that are troubling you is priceless.

Here, I might suggest that, rather than a family member, you find a friend who is willing to be your "ventee." Spouses, children, or very close personal friends are often struggling as much or more than you might be. My wife certainly struggled more, and still does. I don't vent to her, since that would be counterproductive. Don't add more to what they are already dealing with. Bursts of frustration, anger, and the like are best shared with someone who will just take it and get rid of it for you. This spares those closest to you added stressors, and protects the strength of your already existing relationship. I believe this wisdom to be sound. I will say, however, that Liz simply said after reading this, "For better or worse. You can vent on me if you need to." So there—I guess I've been told. Still, I see the toll venting can take on a loved one, and I encourage you to find another "ventee."

A word of caution: there will come those times when we're just not ready to be a listener, to hear certain kinds of news. We just don't want to hear it as a patient. This is why I believe it is so important to be honestly open. In times like these, if we have developed an honest relationship, we are freed to politely share with them that we are not willing to share at this time about how we are feeling. Without openness, feelings often get hurt or misunderstandings poison an otherwise great relationship. People are simply less likely to take offense when a safe space has been created to deal with just these types of situations. When open and honest dialogue is allowed, much more helping rather than hurting becomes available. It is hard enough to share at times even when willing; we don't need to make it harder by misunderstood good intentions. Finally, a consideration I must address is our life's course. My favorite Bible passage is 1 Corinthians 9:24. In it Paul talks about winning and losing, starting versus finishing. This reflects much of how I view life. So what is my course? How am I to finish? I've already touched on some of my feelings about these matters, but life begs the question, "When I finish, and I will, how is my finish to look? None of us can know the answer to this question, but some of us think we know, or have a better idea than others. I have run enough races by now to know that most times we are surprised by what the finish brings.

Whether I have ever admitted it to anyone or not, the process has made me ask myself, "What if there are fights we're not meant to win—battles it is our destiny to lose—what then? Some will argue that this is just not fair! You have that right. I have not openly discussed the "Why me?" questions. By now you should have your own list set in your mind, but if you don't know by now then you have missed the whole message. So I'll spell it out.

My mission to others, my trust in my Savior, my spiritual growth as someone discontent with stagnation, and MY appointment with my destiny are driving me toward God's mysterious end for me—however that may look. Cancer or not, what a journey! What a magnificent journey!

I know I'm not Jesus, and would never imply otherwise. You may not believe in Jesus, but that's between him and you and that's OK with me. But I want to say that Jesus met his course with meticulous orchestration. He relinquished his life in apparent defeat as his pathway to victory. Death had its day—but Jesus claimed my ETERNITY!

As a younger man I was driven to make requests of God. I would tell him things like: "I want to know you more or better;" "I want to be used;" "I want a mission;" "Please Lord, grow my faith—let me be a witness;" "Let me be me for you."

For a while as I drove to work I would tell God, "This is where I am; this is my field; put me to work today so it is not a day spent worthlessly." I would remind God that he was the one who said, "The harvest is ready but the workers are few." I would remind him that it was he who put me here, who made me who I am, and if I can't do some good here, then put me where I can. If the only outcomes of my day are the required tasks associated with this job, and there are no tangible fruits to show for this time other than that, I feel it is a waste of my life.

CLINT SAID IT BEST

"Do you feel lucky, punk? Well, do ya?" What an awesome, unforgettable line. I'd hazard to guess that at least seventy-five percent of the "world's" population knows of that line made famous by Clint Eastwood in the movie Dirty Harry. Staring down the barrel of his .357 magnum he asks, "Well, do you?" What an awesome question. Well, do I? Yes, I do, and not because my tests are still all good. Day to day life is rolling along and running pretty normal, or the new normal anyway.

Honestly speaking, all this cancer junk *comes to mind* a lot. For a moment I was going to say, "I *think* about it a lot," but I don't *think* about it a lot. It does come *to* mind, but over time I have worked out a way that lets it pass *across* my mind but not stop by for a visit. There's a big difference between the two, passing vs. pausing. I am lucky.

I've also learned some powerful lessons on helping and being helped. Sometimes our initial reaction is to reject someone's expression of concern or care. We tell them, "It's not a good time" or, shrug them off with an, "I'm fine." I challenge you to let them in. I hated letting people in at first, and I have "prided" myself on not needing anyone's help. These acts too have demonstrated my weakness, rather than my strength.

Things come into true perspective when the phone rings, and it's the doctor's office. Things once thought important aren't so important any more. Passions change. Your views about work or family can become flipped into the order they should have been in all along. I do feel lucky. And as part of these new discoveries true friends are discovered, real friends. Some we have known all along, thank goodness. Some we knew all along really turn out to be not so friend-like. Funny how life can be flipped on its head—funny how our head flips. Yes, oh yes, I do feel lucky!

So here's the kicker. So maybe this is it. This disease is my answer to prayer. Who among us has not wanted to feel useful? Who has not wanted to find meaning in their life? For those of you who believe, who has not wanted to see their faith grow or sought a more intimate relationship with our Savior? I prayed, asked, or begged for all of those things! I wanted them then; I want them still. I have always wanted a way to be all in! From here it looks like God heard every word, and took it to heart. So I am who I prayed I would become, or I am who He wanted me to become all along. I am who I am, evolving. It's still an adventure, and I'm right on course, thank God.

POSTSCRIPT

Today I got one of those calls again. Last week I went in for my second follow-up chest CT to check on those "new" lung nodules. Today Ginger asked me if I had ever seen a pulmonologist (lung expert). "Nope" I told her. She went on to say, "Well, Dr. Frank would like you to see Dr. Miller here at Loyola. You have had stable nodules all along, but now you have some new small ones, and he wants him to look at them to see what's going on."

March 10th was the office visit. It went much like the phone call. They found two new nodules in my left lung. After the visit was concluded I headed out to the appointment desk. I scheduled an appointment with the pulmonologist for March 22.

So here we are, six and a half years of being in the clear, and now I'm probably looking at a tissue biopsy. I'm also back to CT and doctor visits on a three-month schedule. What a flashback; right back to square one. No tidy conclusion, but after all, it isn't the movies.

Reactions to this turn of events have been interesting. Many have offered bewildered looks when they hear me talk like this. Most just say they heard about the "bad news." Coworkers would tell you I got quiet at the news, or appeared worried at the call. I did get quiet. You can't help but wonder.

Times like these do have a way of taking over your mind.

So for now it's like a flash back to the beginning. In fact, it feels just as the beginning did, especially when they said, "Oh, I'm sure it'll be nothing." But your gut tells you otherwise. If it was really nothing, then why are we adding unexpected appointments, and doctors, and tests? But instead I kept silent and followed the new orders. More calling, more waiting, more interruptions in life, or *are they*? Everything else gets put on hold while you wait for return calls. This just means that when you're trying to do life you must focus harder to get things accomplished, or just resign yourself to the truth that reminds that more time will just have to be sacrificed on the altar of waiting. My mind tends to jump around during these times. It's very frustrating, still. I have often heard it said, "Patience is a virtue." Maybe.

If all this has taught me anything critical to my very living it is this: I have come to understand that cancer was always to be as much a part of my life as has life with God and any of the other days and events before and after cancer. God was not surprised by this new diagnosis. He was not caught off guard. By his grace alone I too am not surprised, or caught off guard. Cancer was never meant to be a stroke of bad luck; cancer has brought God and me to a place that we never would have shared otherwise. The culmination of these last six and half years has taught me that life will always be full of challenges to living, to living out life faithfully. Soon I'll find out if these newly discovered nodules are cancerous. When I asked the doctor what the follow-up *treatment* (notice I said "treatment") for lung nodules was, he said, "Chemo." Sometimes short and sweet is a whole lot better than long and drawn out.

So here it is, about a week or so later. Liz and I have seen Dr. Miller. He had reviewed my lung CT and concluded that the infamous new nodules may not even exist. I guess because it is an image of a series of dissections, anomalies can pop up that aren't really there. He said the only way to know for sure would be to cut me open, and he wasn't willing to do that. He said they are just too small to worry about. I looked at Liz, and she at me. This was just the doctor's visit both of us had been praying for. Phew. That was that. Before I left, I thanked both the doctor and his intern for their time, and said, "Don't take this the wrong way, but I hope never to see either of you ever again." Everybody smiled, we shook hands, and then Liz and I walked out.

To date I am still good. To date I am still getting CT scans, but Dr. Frank said we would switch to chest x-rays after my next visit set for December of 2011.

✱ ✱ ✱

So there you have it. I'm glad I'm in good hands. I'm glad I don't have to try to carry the whole load. And even though it may at times feel like the beginning all over again, it's NOT! I am not the same Guy. I am stronger and healthier than ever, mentally and spiritually. There is much said about finding "the cure." I know that countless armies of folks are tirelessly working everyday to find "the cure," and who can blame them.

But what if CANCER is meant *to be* the CURE! Many of the things that plagued me for years were only cured because of this journey with cancer. I would not be the man I am, and I would not be the man of faith that I am, if not for cancer. So while they seek, I've found. While they are hopeful, I am hope-filled. I don't wonder if "the cure" is out there, because I have found it!

Whether you want to admit it or not, we will all die from something. It's just a matter of when, not if. The question is— are you ready? For me, Jesus became the *cure* that gives me Life and Peace, and Victory even over the grip of Death himself!

About the Author

* * *

So who am I? I can tell you what I've done; I've been a cabinetmaker, dental technician, and supervisor for a Public Works facility. But who am I really? In my search to know this I can tell you I attained three college degrees, culminating in a Master of Divinity from Northern Seminary. But disease cares little about these. Instead, I offer that I am just a Guy in the act of Living! I have been blessed by my wife Liz of 27 years and counting, and our son Dan. Together we live in Naperville, IL, and share our lives with many dear friends.